EXERCISE IS FUN

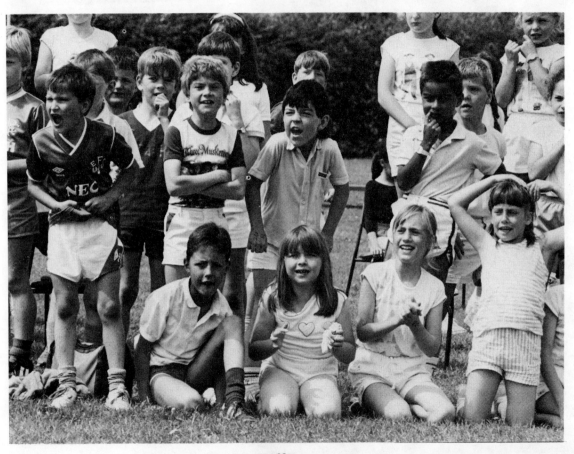

foulsham educational

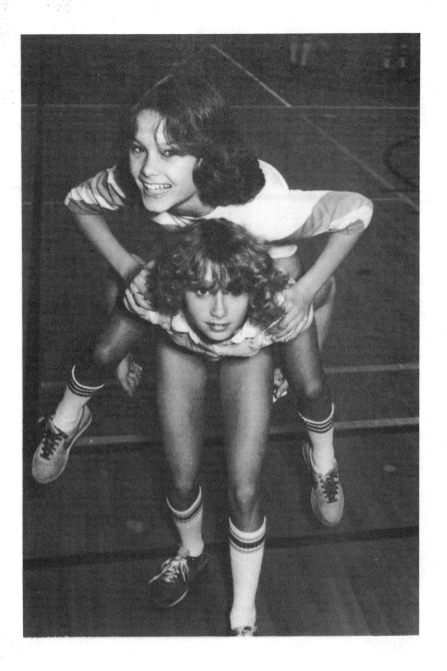

This book is dedicated to Laura Jane, Heather, and Stefan Steen, for their inspiration.

foulsham

Yeovil Road, Slough, Berkshire SL1 4JH

ISBN 0-572-01650-6

Printed in Great Britain by
St Edmundsbury Press Limited, Bury St Edmunds, Suffolk

The author would like to thank Cassie Gairdner for her help in taking the photographs. Additional photographs on pages 1, 4, 7, 51, 67, 96, 110 & 122 by Alan L. Edwards.

Contents

3. New Fun in Old Games / 51

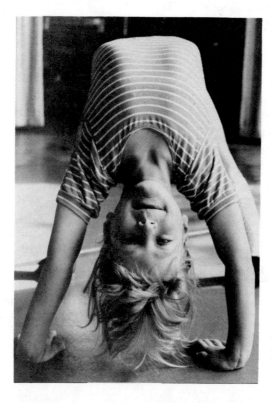

4. Aerobic Races and Relays / 78

5. Run For Fun / 92

6. Aerobic Challenges / 104

7. How Fit Are You / 122

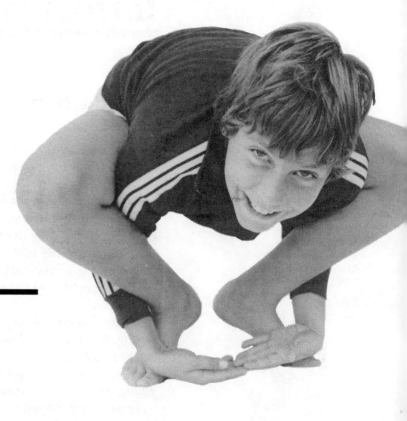

Introduction

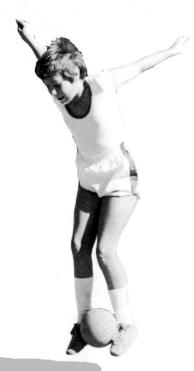

Introduction

In this book, teachers will find a large variety of interesting ways to motivate children to take up cardio-respiratory exercises, and find rewarding diversions from regular training routines. Parents will also discover ways to encourage fitness in their children; and young people themselves will find that the following games and exercises not only have good personal health and fitness value, but are also lots of fun.

Many traditional exercises are repitious and boring. It requires a dedicated parent or teacher and an unusual child to do rigorous daily exercises. To make fitness attractive to all young people, more than games and exercises have been developed for this book. Many are brand new. Some of them will be familiar to readers but their special aerobic benefits may be unexpected. Some are suitable for individuals, others are best for groups, large or small. Adults as well as children will enjoy many of them.

Fitness is vital. Everybody knows that by now. Physical fitness seems to improve health, reduce stress and improve concentration. In children it also promotes correct growth and development.

It's a myth that children are naturally active. The average child watches television three hours a day, and is being raised in a world of electronic gadgetry where one of the greatest tests of strength is to open the refrigerator door. It is said that the average youngster's fitness begins to decline at age five, with the result that by the time she or he is a teenager, the potential for useful physical and mental work has been drastically reduced.

Depending, of course, on the measurement criteria, up to three quarters of the country's school population could be described as 'unfit'. Over the past few years physical education has been a neglected area in schools, either because of a lack of resources, teachers, or time — or just general apathy. The advent of a

National Curriculum for schools to follow should encourage a welcome reversal of this trend.

Over the past decade the average primary school child received only sixty minutes of physical education each week, and much of that time was spent changing clothes, listening to instructions, waiting for a turn, and playing non-fitness games.

Ideally, sixty minutes each *day* should be set aside for physical education.

With the advent of compulsory physical education on a structured basis in schools, the need for an ideas book such as this will be paramount, not only as a resource use for specialist teachers, but also as a useful reference for non-specialist teachers who may feel at a loss when it comes to planning useful, varied, daily fitness programmes.

Health researchers have found that an alarming number of children, even six-year-olds, already possess more than one coronary risk factor such as obesity, low work capacity, or high levels of dangerous fats in the blood. One study of active youngsters identified the most common risk factor in seven to twelve-year-olds as obesity. Because they tend to move more slowly, fat children can become discouraged when playing with thinner children. Ironically, the overweight children who are most in need of exercise are often the ones who are ignored because they can't keep up and let the side down. Many of the games in this book are non-competitive, which means they're ideal for informal fitness routines with mixed-fitness groups including obese children.

The heart of an average adult beats seventy-two times each minutes. The average heart will beat 4.320 times every hour; 104,000 times every day; 38 million times each year and 2.7 billion times in the average lifespan of seventy years, with no time off! It's "heartening" to note that if the resting heart-rate is reduced by regular exercise, say to two thirds of the average rate, the heart will beat 900 million fewer times in a human life. Good mileage!

The number of heart beats multiplied by the volume of blood ejected with each beat is called cardiac output. Regular exercise gradually lowers the resting heart-rate, and increases the per-stroke volume of blood ejected. The heart is a muscle that is itself strengthened by exercise. Having good, clear arteries is also important for the health of the heart muscle, and exercise helps to enlarge the coronary arteries and develops extra vessels around the heart.

Aerobic exercise reduces the possibility of cardio-vascular-pulmonary diseases by building the lungs, vascular system and heart. Aerobic exercises are continuous exercises of moderate intensity, which require a steady flow of oxygen to the working muscles. For example, running at a steady pace in which the heart-rate is not raised above 150 beats per minute is an aerobic exercise. Children may experience muscular and mental fatigue while doing aerobic exercise, but they won't be forced to give up because heart, arteries, veins, air passages and lungs can't provide enough

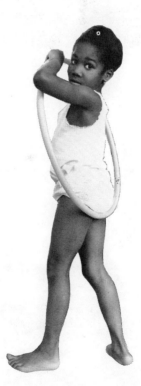

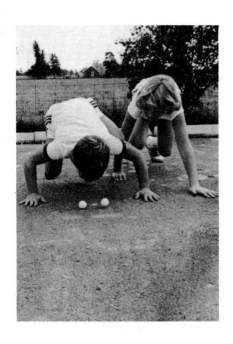

oxygen to the muscles.

Anaerobics, by contrast, means any exercise done with insufficient oxygen. Anaerobic metabolism is the burning of fuel with too little oxygen. This type of exertion uses up glycogen, a complex natural sugar stored mostly in the muscle fibres and liver. Anaerobic energy is released rapidly and lasts only a few moments. A 100 or 200 metre sprinter will perform almost entirely on stores of energy already present in the body, and by the time he or she has completed the event, a substantial 'oxygen debt' will have been built, to be paid back during the rest period following the race. Of course, different exercises involve varying proportions of aerobic and anaerobic metabolism.

'Fitness' is a relative term, but it may be thought of as the long-term ability to perform routine duties with a minimum of fatigue and discomfort, and to be physically and mentally alert to meet and overcome challenges.

Fitness is a way of life and not a two-week enthusiasm for jogging or push-ups. In one way, it's a war against two relentless forces of nature: gravity, which can make the load heavy and rounds the shoulders in old age, and disintegration, which in time destroys everything. To delay the effect of these forces, a fitness programme should contain variety, challenge, and a means of measuring progress. The road to fitness is cluttered with those who break down because they start too fast. Good planning is essential. The goal and plan must be realistically suited to the participant's

abilities: even the best-planned fitness programme is useful only to the people who actually follow it.

A sound programme will emphasise cardio-respiratory activities, tax all muscles (stretching and stressing them to a safe limit), move joints through their full range, reduce adrenal products in the blood, improve balance and coordination, and include activities to release tensions and express emotions. A programme should be progressive in its demands, but should be adapted to suit participants' strengths, weaknesses, likes and dislikes. Activities should be organised in a way that allows more success than failure, and permits tangible improvement in performance.

Most exercises are worthwhile, especially those requiring the use of large muscles for extended periods. No two experiences produce exactly the same effect and no single exercise is adequate to produce complete fitness, although some are better than others.

When planning routines for young people, it's especially important to remember to fit the game to the child, not the child to the game. Teachers must try to put themselves in a child's shoes, where running one kilometre feels like an adult's ten, a football pitch seems far longer than a run round the block, and a basketball hoop looks as high as the sky. It's also important to make allowances for individuality. The group leader who relies totally on team games may be disappointed when some youngsters fail to thrive. Some will "hide" during games because they are shy, lazy, lack the skill, speed and aggression of other children, or are simply day-dreaming. A good child-fitness programme should therefore include both individual and group activities.

The exercises in this book have been designed and chosen because they are aerobically beneficial, varied, suitable for children in physical terms, and also appealing to children in terms of interest and entertainment. Selecting from the activities here will provide a useful and constructive base upon which to build a structured programme of physical education for children of all ages.

The National Curriculum for England and Wales in physical education for ages 5 to 16 identifies the "provision of physical education and recreation of young people".

This book goes a long way to providing a considerable number of options from which a teacher can select in composing a programme for all key stages and attainment levels covering exercise, athletic activities, games, gymnastic activities, outdoor, adventurous and water-based activities.

Exercise Selection Grid	
INDIVIDUALS	Page No. 1-21; 36; 39-40; 46-48; 53; 56; 62; 64; 67; 79-81; 96; 103; 105-6; 116-121; 123-125
DOUBLES	Page No. 23-25; 41-43; 49; 65; 81; 91; 106
GROUPS OR TEAMS	Page No. 27-33; 35-37; 41; 44-45; 47; 49-50; 52; 54; 56; 58-62; 65-66; 68-77; 82-91; 94-103; 108-115

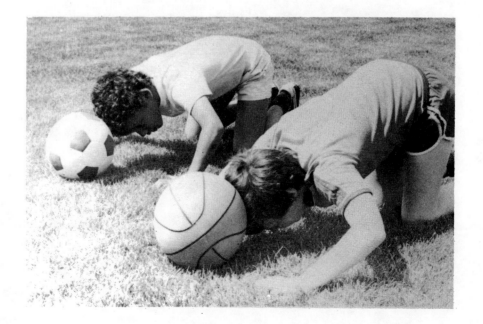

CHAPTER 1

Exercises

Exercises heat the body from the inside out, enabling it to go through a full range of motions without pain or discomfort, and raising the heart-rate and blood flow to the muscles in readiness for heavier activities.

Don't hurry through warm-up exercises. Warm-ups are egalitarian and non-competitive, and provide time for the group leader to talk briefly with each participant, especially those who need special attention and encouragement. If time is short, choose exercises that use the big muscles in the body, such as the All Over Stretch, instead of those that work exclusively on small isolated parts of the body. Children should do exercises slowly and smoothly, never holding their breath for more than a few seconds. Warm-ups should last between 10 and 15 minutes.

Exercises for Individuals

DOUBLE LEG THRUSTS

Assume a full push-up position. Draw both feet forward, bending knees tightly under chest, then thrust legs together back to the starting position. Do this exercise during a count of 20, take a break, then do two more sets of the same length. One difficult alternative, calling for considerable flexibility, is to keep legs straight throughout the exercise. Hips must be raised high, while feet are pulled as close as possible to hands.

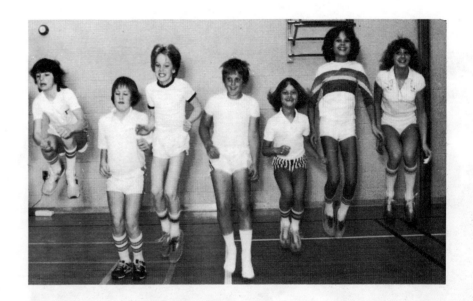

DOWN AND OUT

From a standing position, quickly crouch and place both hands on floor just in front of feet. With arms straight, thrust feet backwards to assume a push-up position. Immediately resume crouch and then stand. Participants should do one Down and Out for each year of their age.

KNEE TUCK JUMPS

Jump up and down on the spot. Gradually, while jumping, draw knees higher and higher until they almost touch chest. Then gradually lower knees with each jump. This is a strenuous exercise, so start with only two or three repetitions. As fitness improves, increase the number of repetitions, with rests in between.

11

GROUND LOOPS

Place one hand on the ground with arm straight. Keeping body as straight as possible, walk round hand in a circle. Switch hands and walk in the opposite direction.

COMPASS CIRCLES

Compass Circles are particularly useful for helping improve motor skills. In each variation of Compass Circles, the hands remain in the centre of the compass, the body forms the compass needle, and the feet describe the circle.

Assume a push-up position, keeping arms and body as straight as possible. With hands on the same spot, walk round sideways in a circle. Allow hands to slide round freely while turning. Now walk in the opposite direction. Repeat twice.

In the same position, repeat the exercise but keep feet together, making circles with a sideways hopping motion.

Try each of these exercises again in a stomach-up position, crab-style.

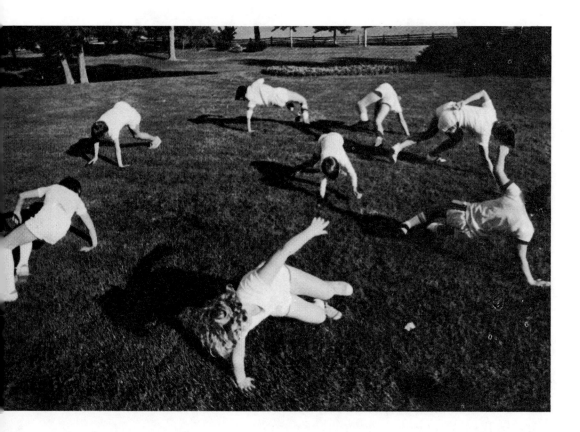

HOOP-DE-HOOP

Put a hoop on the floor. *Rhythmically* (count time, or perform this exercise to music), hop on both feet in and out of the hoop. Hop in and out on right foot, then on left foot.

Hopping in and out on both feet, travel around the hoop. Repeat the exercise on right foot only, then on left. Go backwards. Try going backwards on one foot!

KNEE SLAPS

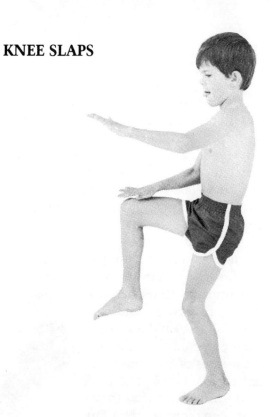

Run on the spot. Keep hands, palms down, at waist level. Lift knees high enough to slap hands.

LEG EXCHANGES

With legs split fore and aft and arms bent in running position, quickly reverse the position of feet, and continue the exchanges at a steady pace. Maintain the wide spacing of feet and avoid moving body up and down.

MULE KICK

Standing, bend forward, palms on the ground 50 cm in front of toes, so that body forms a high bridge. Put weight on hands and spring off both feet so heels gently touch the buttocks and return to the same place on the ground. Repeat ten times.

SQUATS

Stand with feet comfortably apart, arms at sides. Keeping heels flat on floor and swinging arms forward, lower body until thighs are parallel to floor. Stand up. This is one complete Squat. Each knee-bend counts as one repetition.

Try squatting on one leg only, or rise so fast that feet leave the ground in a Jump Squat. The deeper the crouch, the greater the effort.

Squats are excellent aerobic and leg-strengthening exercises. One variation that is especially good for flexibility and balance is the Sideways Squat. Squat and touch the outside of right heel with both hands, stand up tall, then squat to touch both hands on left heel.

13

ONE-LEGGED SQUAT

Standing, hold left foot in left hand behind buttocks, lower left knee onto a mat, then return to starting position. Most people will discover that this is a challenging exercise. For this reason, make certain the knee touches down on a soft surface. If necessary, hold onto a partner's hand or the wall during the exercise. Try only one squat with each leg at first. As fitness improves, more repetitions may be attempted.

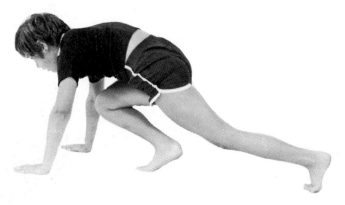

STATIONARY STARTS

Assume a full push-up position. Without moving hands and keeping buttocks as low as possible, begin switching legs. Bring the knee of the front leg close up under chest and stretch out the back leg, then change legs. Count to 20 while doing this exercise, rest, then do two more sets of the same length. Try not to let back sag when back leg is fully extended.

STEP-UPS

This is one of the few exercises in this section which requires apparatus. A chair, stairs, or a low beam will do. The exercise is simple: step on and off the beam. It doesn't really matter whether the lead leg alternates or one leg leads continuously for one minute and the other for the next minute. The aerobic benefit is derived from the height of the step, the technique (stand tall at the top of the Step-ups), and the frequency and duration of Step-ups.

The Step-up is the most simple of three basic exercises (the others are cycling and running on a treadmill) used in tests to measure oxygen-uptake capacities. Older participants (11-15 years) may want to take their pulse immediately after two minutes of Step-ups on a 40 cm high step or bench, and then again two minutes later after they have rested. They can compare their pulses with each other. The figures will show that the heart-rate increases with work and decreases with a post-work rest. Regular aerobic exercise should reduce the time it takes for the heart-rate to return to normal after exertion, and also lower the resting pulse.

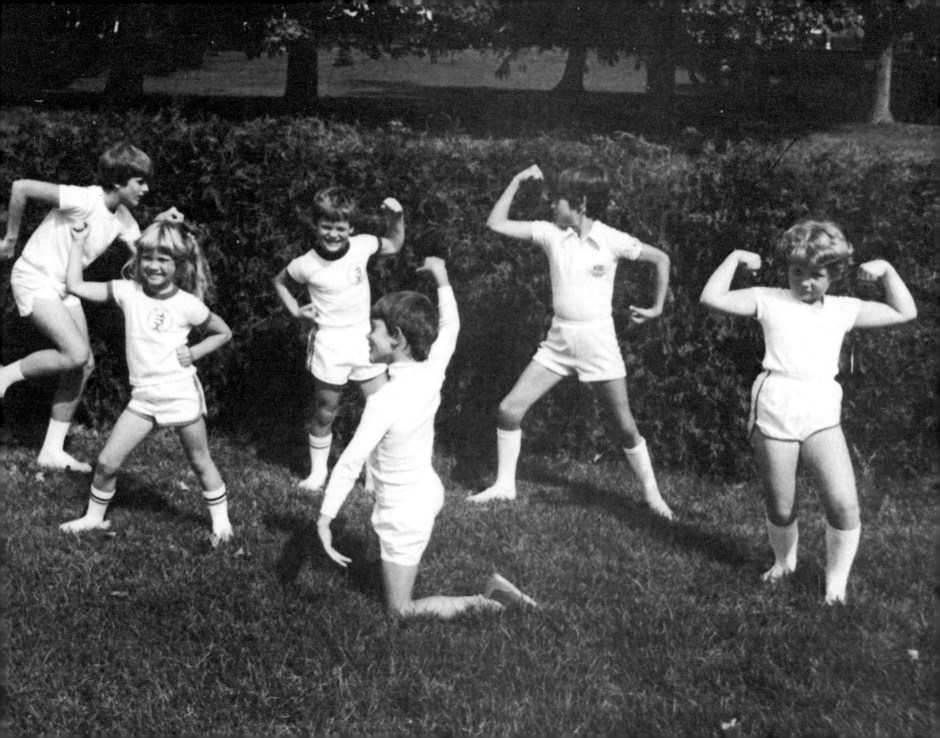

POSES

Ask players to pretend they are muscular body builders posing in a contest. They will laugh while trying out various poses. Present a 'body beautiful' award to the player who would otherwise receive too little attention.

Although these aren't aerobic exercises, they add fun to a warm-up session and build players' strength and awareness of their musculature. Placing youngsters in statice poses in which muscles are tightened also helps them learn various sports skills. For instance, have them 'freeze' in the perfect racquet-ready position of a tennis or squash player.
Squeeze the muscles during each pose only for a count of five.

STRADDLE HOPS

Stand with feet on either side of a low, narrow, stable bench or other raised object 10-40 cm high. Hop onto it, stand tall, then return to the starting position and repeat. This exercise, of course, can be made easy or difficult, depending on the height of the bench, and the frequency and duration of the hops.

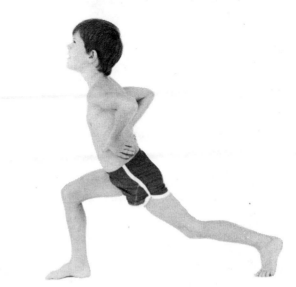

LUNGE

Stand with feet together and hands on hips. Take a mighty long step, bending knee to a right angle. Keep body upright with weight over lead leg. Push back to starting position and repeat with the other leg. Each lunge is a repetition. Do ten repetitions with each leg.

TWISTER

Stand with hands behind head. Raise one knee to meet opposite elbow. Return to start position. Repeat with the opposite knee and elbow. Each elbow-knee touch is one repetition. This exercise can also be performed in a sit-up position. Continue repeating this exercise while you count to 30.

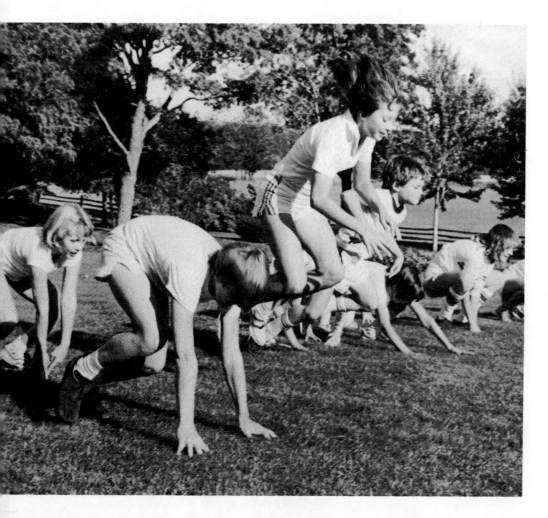

In a crouch, hands on floor (arms either inside or outside the thighs), spring forward, resume the crouch position, then leap again. Because of the temptation to 'cheat' by raising the body higher and higher with each successive leap, Frog Hops aren't recommended for races and relays. To encourage good form offer a reward to the frog with the best technique.

PUSH-UPS

Trouble with Push-ups? Try one of these variations:

Instead of lying face down on floor, place feet on floor and rest hands on a low beam or chair. As long as feet and legs are lower than head and chest, Push-ups will be easier. Practise doing them this way; as strength increases, normal Push-ups will seem easier.

Or, stand with palms of hands against a wall and lean forward so that arms are bent. Push till arms are straight, then lean again and repeat.

On the other hand, if ordinary Push-ups present no problem, make them more difficult by keeping arms and chest *below* the level of legs. Doing Push-ups while resting feet on a beam or chair will develop good arm, shoulder and chest strength. To develop chest power, spread hands wide apart. For strengthening the triceps (back of upper arm) keep hands close together.

FROG HOPS

Properly executed, Frog Hops are strenuous exercises for the cardio-respiratory system and the large muscles of the legs and back.

17

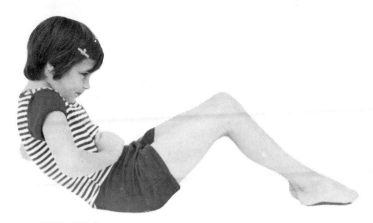

ROLL UP AND TUCK

Lie on back, with arms stretched out beyond head and hands touching. Swing arms forward in a sit-up motion and at the same time pull knees to chest. Touch toes and unfold. Six- to eight-year-olds may find this exercise difficult.

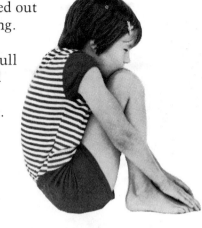

SIT-UPS

Many children find ordinary bent-knee Sit-ups with hands behind heads difficult. To help, anchor feet under a partner or some object such as a low bench, or place hands on stomachs during sit-ups. If an incline-board or sloping ground is available, point feet down the slope.

For older children, variations of this useful exercise include Twisting Sit-ups (alternating left elbow to right knee and right elbow to left knee), Half Sit-ups (sit up only until back is clear of floor and toes are visible), and Sit-up and Stretch (with straight legs, touch toes, but do it slowly).

TWO-POINT CROUCH

Crouch down and place hands on ground between feet, about 50 cm apart. Braced on slightly bent arms, rock forward allowing feet to leave ground. Hold for a count of five, relax, and repeat.

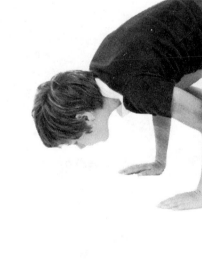

WALL WALK

Start in arched push-up position with feet against base of a wall and head pointing away from wall. In bare feet or clean shoes, walk up the wall with small steps, without moving hands, until handstand position is achieved, then walk down wall again.

ALL OVER STRETCH

Assume a push-up position, fingers pointing straight ahead. Keeping arms straight, drop pelvis close to floor and look straight up. Hold this position for a count of three, then, without moving hands or feet, force hips high and look back at feet. Hold for another count of three.

An arching movement followed by a bridging movement is one repetition. Placing feet against wall will prevent slipping. Six- to eight-year-olds may find this excellent stretching exercise difficult.

IMITATIONS

Have players pretend they are something that can move swiftly — a river, the wind, rain, motor cycle, animal, airplane, train, bird, lorry or fish. They should move in slow motion first, then powerfully, finally making a noise like whatever it is they are pretending to be.

FLOOR HIP STRETCH

Assume a push-up position supported on only one arm. With arm and body straight, look straight ahead. Without bending elbow of supporting arm, let hips sag to floor. Hold this position for a count of three, return to the start position and repeat the exercise three times on each arm.

LEAN A LITTLE

Keeping heels on floor throughout the exercise, lean at a slight angle against a wall, facing the wall and touching it with hands. Keep arms straight. Hold for a count of 15, then slide back 30 cm and count to 15 again. Repeat four times with feet farther from the wall each time.

GOIN' NOWHERE

Assume push-up position with hands directly below shoulders. Without moving hands take small steps forward until toes touch wrists. Walk back to starting position. Repeat three times.

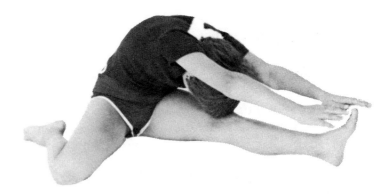

HURDLE STRETCH

Sitting on floor, stretch right leg straight ahead and tuck left heel close to left buttock. Reach with both hands toward right foot, bringing forehead close to knee. Hold this stretch for a count of three, return to starting position, and repeat stretch three times. Change position so left leg is stretched straight ahead, and repeat routine.

Optional stretches in this hurdle position include pulling head to bent knee and also lying back to touch back of head on floor.

HIGH HURDLE STRETCH

Standing, place heel of straight right leg on railing or similar support at hip height. Reach with both hands towards raised foot, bringing head close to knee. Hold for a count of three, return to starting position, relax and repeat five times. Repeat routine with left leg raised. One variation is to place heel of straight right leg on railing and reach towards foot of straight left leg.

STRETCH AND SLOUCH

Standing, join hands on top of head. Breathe deeply and stretch both arms, hands still clasped together, high overhead. Tilt head back and lift chest for a count of five, then exhale in a long, easy sigh, letting hands fall apart at sides. Let head and shoulders sag forward and bend knees slightly. Relax and let tension flow out of the body. Remain in the slouch for a count of five, then repeat entire exercise.

SWIVEL HIPS

Standing with feet comfortably apart, slowly rotate hips in largest possible circle, keeping head and feet still. Rotate in one direction for a count of 20, then change direction and count to 20 again.

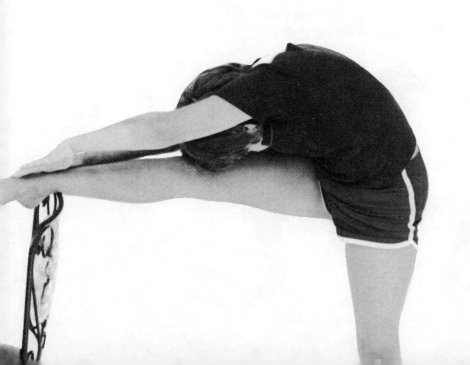

21

Exercises for Partners

DON'T KICK ME

Partners stand back to back, left hands on left knees, and right hands reaching between legs to join in hand-to-hand grip. One partner swings right leg over partner's back and then back to the starting position. The other partner does the same. Each partner does the exercise three times with right leg and three with left.

LOTS OF SQUATS

Partners stand face to face, hold hands, and together do 15 Half-squats, or do alternate Squats. Or, stand back to back, link elbows, and squat slowly together.
Do 15 repetitions of each variation.

PARTNER SKI-SITS

Starting seated back to back on the floor, partners push themselves into ski-sit positions, thighs parallel to the floor, and hold them for a count of 20. For fun, try walking about in this ski-sit position.

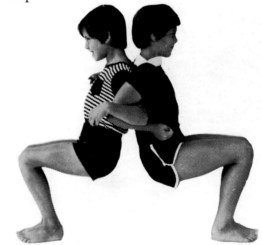

BACK-UP-ME

Partners stand back to back and link arms at
elbows. One leans forward, raising the other off
the ground, and moves forward for a set
distance. Partners then change places so that
the carrier is carried back to the start line.

PARTNER PULL-UPS

Partners sit on floor in bent-knee sit-up
position, facing each other, toe to toe. Grasping
hands, they pull one another to a standing
position then return to the floor. Repeat five
times.

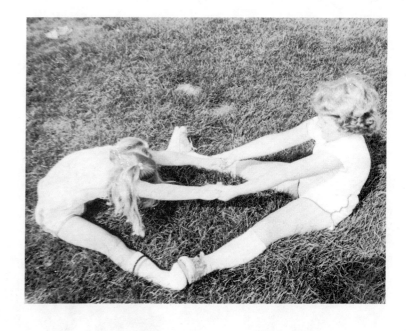

UP THE CREEK WITH A PARTNER

Partners sit on ground facing each other,
holding hands. For first rowing exercise, they
spread feet wide, bracing each other soles
against soles. They then row with long, slow
strokes for 3 separate counts of 30, taking a
10-count rest between spells of rowing.

For the second rowing routine, partners
assume the hurdle stretch position (left leg
straight ahead and right leg tucked under right
buttock, left sole on partner's right knee). Do
same number of sets and repetitions.

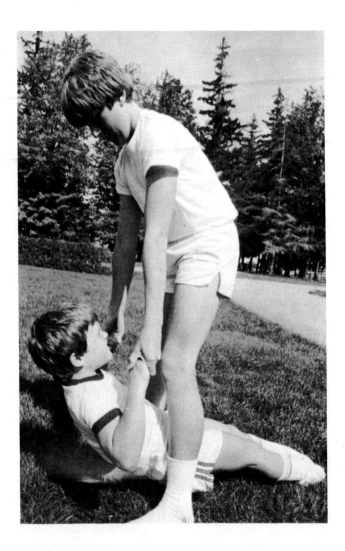

PARTNER CHIN-UPS

In each pair, one partner stands astride and grasps the hands of the other partner, who lies on his or her back on the ground. The partners who are lying down try to pull themselves up as far as possible, then lower themselves back onto the ground. To prevent slipping, the lower partners can brace their feet against a wall.

Each partner should do three sets of five Chin-ups.

PIGGYBACK EXERCISES

Piggybacking is an excellent aerobic and strength exercise, but is not advised for players under nine unless they are unusually strong. It is very important for partners to be around the same size.

Piggyback Walk Have each partner carry the other for a short distance on flat ground or, better still, up a hillside.

Piggyback Step-ups Step on and off a stable bench or low chair, switching places often.

Piggyback Heel-raises The piggyback pair face a wall, leaning slightly towards it. The rider presses hands against the wall for support. The 'horse' raises heels as high off the floor as possible and lowers them, repeating 5 to 15 times before switching partners.

Piggyback Squats In the same position as for Piggyback Heel-raises, the 'horse' lowers body, keeping trunk upright, to a one-eighth, one-quarter, or one-half squat position (depending on leg strength). Partner should be raised and lowered 3 to 12 times, then partners should switch places. Back injuries can be caused if the 'horse' bends over. To keep the back straight, the 'horse' should focus on an object above eye level.

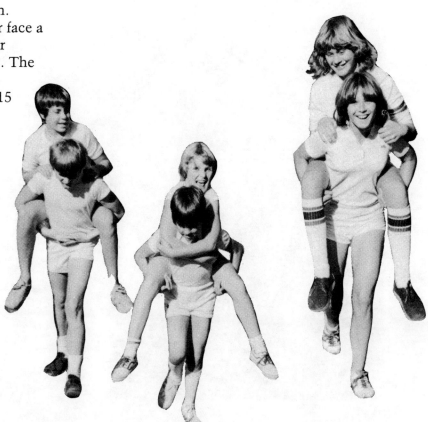

CHAPTER 2
Aerobic Games

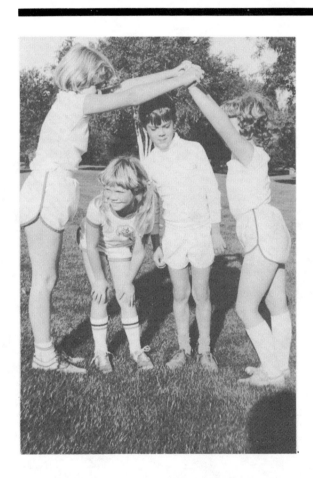

CAPTURE THE FLAG

This game is more effectively played outdoors than in a gymnasium. Mark out a playing area like the one in the diagram. Proper boundaries, marked with cones, white lines or old clothing, will reduce confusion and disputes. The size of the playing area should be based on the number of players and available space. Obstacles such as trees, small hills, and ditches will add interest.

Divide the group into two teams of equal numbers. Each team belongs in one territory. Players are safe while in their own territory, but may be tagged in enemy territory. The object of the game is to capture a flag (a shirt or other piece of clothing) from the opponents' half of the field without the thief being tagged. If the thief is tagged, the flag must be returned and the thief sent to prison. The game is ended when the first flag is successfully captured and placed in the centre of the thief's team's flag circle.

Players are safe while they are in opposing team's flag circle; players may not enter their own flag circle. Any player tagged within the opponents' territory (except the flag circle) must go directly to jail. Prisoners can be freed from jail if a team-mate penetrates enemy territory and runs through the jail circle. Freed players can reach safety by running untagged to their own territory or the opponents' flag circle.

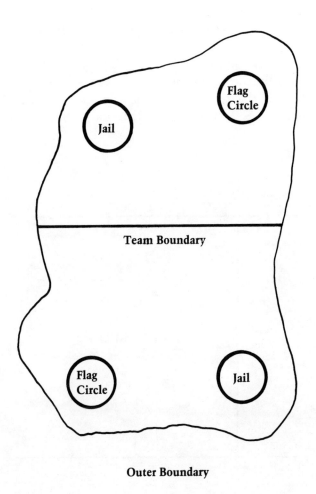

Team Boundary

Outer Boundary

BULLDOGS

This traditional game honours the courage and determination of those muscular, broad-faced little beasts, the bulldogs.

Using any easily visible objects, such as shirts or shoes, mark off the boundaries of a rectangle with safe zones at each end. The size will depend on the number and age of the players.

Select the first bulldog — the player who stands in the centre of the rectangle — and place all the remaining players in one of the safe zones. When the group leader shouts 'Bulldogs!' the players must run to the safe zone at the other end and try to avoid being tagged by the bulldog on the way. A tagged player becomes a bulldog and must stay in the centre of the rectangle to try and tag others on subsequent charges. A bulldog can tag only one player each charge. The winner is the last player to be tagged. He or she becomes the solo bulldog to start the next game.

A mere touch on any part of the body is a tag. Tackling and lifting a captured player off the ground are not allowed. Any player who steps outside the sidelines is automatically a bulldog.

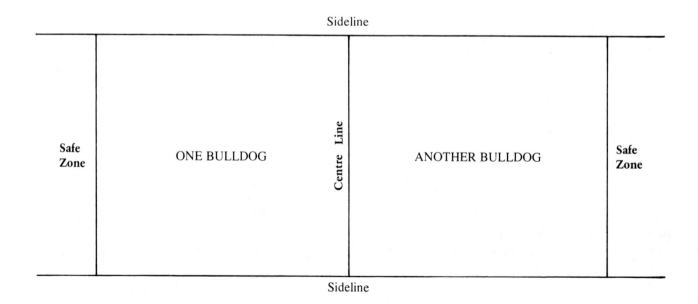

28

SOME BULLDOGS VARIATIONS

- Playing bulldogs up and down a hillside, or having all players working as piggyback pairs (not recommended for youngsters under nine) increases the difficulty, aerobic value and fun.
- Have the bulldogs hold hands, the chain getting longer and more imposing with each run.
- Select every third player to be a bulldog, and place them in the centre of the playing area. The group leader then calls out the method the players are to use to get to the other end of the rectangle, for example hopping on one foot, crab walk or bear walk. A player who is tagged immediately becomes a bulldog while the player who made the tag is free to continue to the safe zone. When all eligible players have reached the safe zone, the group leader calls out another type of movement and the game continues.
- Divide the rectangle into two equal parts, with the centre line parallel to the safe zone lines. Place a bulldog in each section. To remain free, a runner will have to pass untagged through two bulldog territories. If tagged, the runner becomes a bulldog in the area where he or she was tagged. The most populous area when all the players have been tagged is the winner.

SCRAMBLE

Print numbers on as many tennis or similar balls as there are players in the group and assign a number to each player. Scatter the balls in a big gymnasium. At the signal, have the players try to find the ball with their number on it. A player who picks up the wrong ball may throw it anywhere in the gymnasium before proceeding to find his or her own. As players find their own balls, they withdraw from the game, but no player is obliged to pick up his or her own ball if it is more fun to continue dispersing others. Put a 60 or 90 second time limit on each Scramble. After a short rest, gather all the balls and repeat.

Scramble can also be played as a team event. Divide the group into two or more teams. The team to finish first or gather the most balls in 60 to 90 seconds is the winner. Players, of course, will help team-mates find their balls and hinder opponents from locating theirs.

Scramble can also be played in a pool. Print numbers on corks, small blocks of wood, closed plastic bottles, tennis balls — anything that floats and can be numbered. Objects may not be thrown outside the pool.

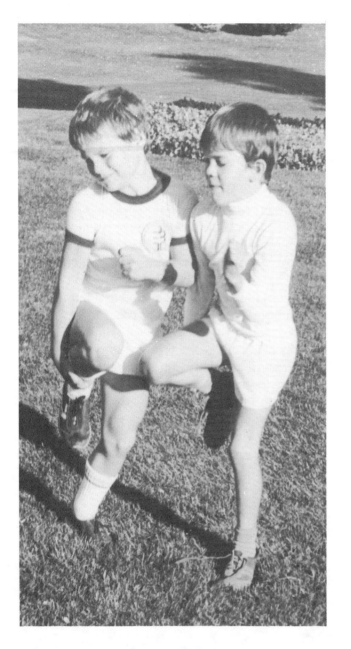

FLAMINGOES

Flamingoes look like gentle birds, but there's nothing gentle about this game, in which players are disguised as flamingoes. Draw a circle on the ground large enough to contain the entire group. Each bird is to raise one leg and grasp the foot. The other hand can't be used to grasp, push or pull other players during the game. The object is to bump others from the circle, or force them to put a second foot down. Any bird who puts down a second foot or is bumped out of the circle must run two laps of the gymnasium (or once around the track) before being readmitted to the circle. After two minutes, no re-entries are permitted. The last remaining bird in the circle is the Fabulous Flamingo.

One excellent variation is to draw a series of small circles, or make a row of hula hoops, equal to the number of flamingoes. They should be 1-2 m apart. Once a bird has been evicted from the large circle, he or she hops to the first small one and has a bumping-contest with its occupant for the right to possess it. The loser hops to the next circle, and so on down the row until all the circles are occupied. No penalties for cooperative birds who agree to share their circle. (This could lead to another game, 'How Many Flamingoes Can Stand on One Leg Inside a Hula Hoop?', but this wouldn't be aerobic.)

Try playing Flamingoes in teams. Divide the group into two or more teams, using coloured vests or bands to distinguish them. The victorious flock is the one with the most birds left in the circle after one minute of bumping.

In the Flamingo Charge, two teams face each other across a battlefield 20 m long. At the signal, the groups advance towards one another. The object is to bump other birds onto two feet. Any bird with both feet down must withdraw from the playing area without interfering with others. The flock with the most birds successfully crossing the battlefield is the winner.

HANGAR FLYING

In this indoor game, the last player to get his entire body off the floor for a count of ten will lose his or her pilot's licence. At the sound of the group leader's whistle, players scramble for ropes, parallel bars, the frame behind the baskets, wall bars or other nearby apparatus. At another whistle, players 'land,' taxi (jog) for two laps, then get back on the runway to take off for a different 'flying' place.

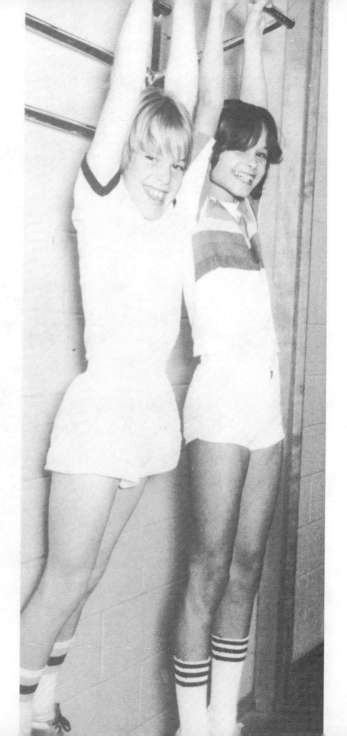

31

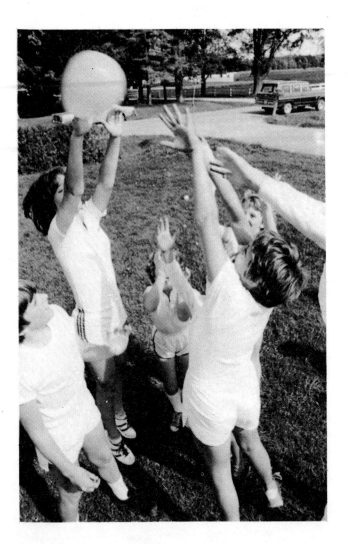

LOONY BALL

This game, played with a large balloon, is fun for all ages. It can be played outdoors on windless days. A goal is scored when the balloon crosses an outdoor goal line (the playing area can be almost any size) or touches against the end walls of a gymnasium. The balloon can only be batted with a single hand. It must not be carried or kicked. If, in the referee's opinion, the balloon is deliberately burst, a goal is awarded to the other team. Choose two teams of three to ten players. The referee tosses up the balloon at the centre line at the beginning of the game and after each goal. Several games can be played on the same area at the same time. For instance, divide a large mixed group into two girls' and two boys' teams.

SCURRY

In this simple game for six to eight-year-olds, scatter bean bags around the gym floor inside a running track. There should be the same number of bags as players. Players run around the loop until a whistle blows or the music stops, when they each run to a bean bag. As they run, the group leader tells them how to touch the bag . . . with right foot, left foot, right knee, left knee, index finger, forehead, back of head, left elbow, right elbow, shoulder, nose, left ear, right ear, chin. When the whistle blows a second time, players begin running around the loop again and the game continues.

KEEPERS WEEPERS

In this simple game possession is everything. It may turn out that the keepers are leapers and the losers are sleepers as well as weepers.

The game is best for a small group, say six to ten players. Have one team wear vests or in some way distinguish themselves. As in man-to-man basketball, break the group into pairs, with a member of each team in each pair. Mark out a small playing area.

The object is to keep a ball, shoe or other object away from the other team. No physical contact is permitted. If a player doesn't pass the ball-object within a count of three, the referee should hand it to the other team. If it's necessary to keep score, each completed pass can be counted as one point. An interception counts for no points.

Players may run with the object or dribble it. When it is passed it must momentarily be free of all hands; that is, it can't be handed off. In the event of hand-off, dropped or incompleted pass, or if the ball carrier runs out of bounds, the referee should hand the object over to the other team.

SOME KEEPERS WEEPERS VARIATIONS

- Every pass must be bounced.
- Play with a football, allowing no arm or hand contact.
- Play with hockey sticks.
- Play piggyback.
- Pass with only one hand; even catch with only one hand.
- Play with a medicine ball.
- To speed up the game, try this: if a player with the ball is tagged by an opponent, the ball-object is turned over to that opponent.
- Place half the pairs on each side on a 2-6 m wide no-man's land. Each pass must be made across the strip; no player may step into it.

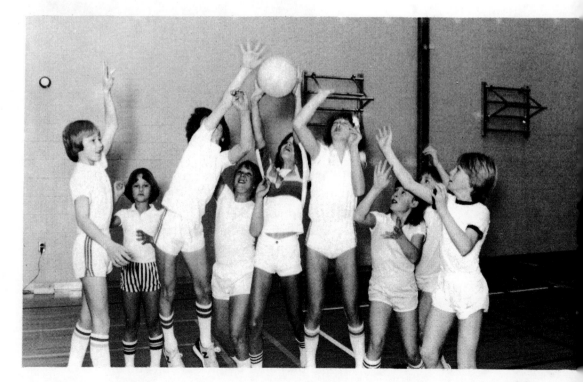

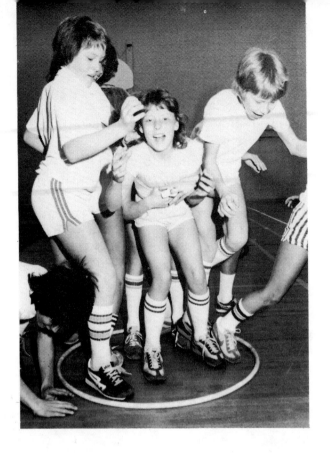

MUSICAL HOOPS

Use cone markers or shirts to mark an oval 80 m track indoors or outdoors. Place hula hoops in a row inside the track, one fewer hoops than total number of players. Instruct players to run around the track, if possible while music plays. When the music stops or a whistle is blown, players rush to occupy a hoop each. Instead of eliminating the player without a hoop, have him or her jump in a hoop with a partner. Start the players off running again.

Remove a hoop each time the music plays, so that eventually all players will be straining to get a foot, toe or finger in the one remaining hoop.

RETRIEVER TRIALS

Assign each player some personal territory, such as a hula hoop placed on the ground, all properties to be clustered at one end of a field or gymnasium. On the floor scatter objects such as bean bags or balls — anything light enough to be carried, and found in abundance in a gymnasium equipment room. The players, at the sound of a whistle, must touch two side walls, then pick up one object and return it to their territory. They must continue this game — touching two walls for each object — until all objects are claimed. The player with the most objects is the Top Dog.

Special recognition could be given to the player of each age group and sex who retrieves the greatest number of objects, and to those who gather the greatest variety. One object could have a special marking, hidden from general view, for which a special prize could be given.

Outdoors, the objects can be scattered over a wider area so that children can run directly to them without having to touch the walls.

After the first game, ask the players to scatter the objects in readiness for the second trial.

RUN THE GAUNTLET

Run the Gauntlet is ideal for a group of 20 to 36 players aged 6 to 15 years. Begin by dividing the group into two teams of equal numbers. Have the players of one team form two rows, spaced evenly along an 8 m wide corridor marked with pylons. Provide each player of this team with a rubber utility ball or slightly deflated volleyball.

The other team starts at one end of the corridor — it should be 20 m long outdoors or almost the length of the gymnasium — and runs to the other end, each runner trying to avoid being hit by balls rolled (not thrown) by the other team. Any player touched by a ball must complete the run but may not run again. The team with the most survivors after three runs each is the winner. Alternatively the game can be played continuously, switching sides (runners to rollers and vice versa) after all the players of one team have been touched by balls.

Anyone struck by a ball above the knee is *not* eliminated from the next run. Similarly, any player touched by a ball outside the corridor or in the end zones is not eliminated.

Change the boundary widths and add or take away utility balls if too many or too few players are running the gauntlet and not being touched by a ball.

One excellent variation of Run the Gauntlet is to place a suitable number of bean bags at the end of the gymnasium opposite the starting area, and give the first team one minute to run the gauntlet to the bags and return them to the starting area. Each player can only take one bag

at a time. Any player struck with a ball while running the gauntlet must return to the starting area and begin again; those carrying a bag while struck must return it to its original place before going empty handed to the starting area. The winning team is the one to collect the greatest number of bags in one minute.

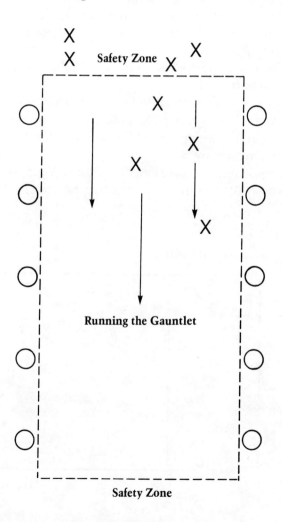

Running the Gauntlet

VICTORY BALL

This game can be played with any number of players, indoors or out. The playing area must have two end zones and room outside the sidelines; the size will depend on the number of players. The object of Victory Ball is to pass a slightly deflated volleyball to a team-mate in the opposing team's end zone. The following rules apply:

- The game begins with a toss-up in the centre, similar to netball.
- No player is allowed to take more than three steps while carrying the ball.
- The ball is moved up and down the playing area mostly by passing.
- A goal can be scored only by a pass. A player who runs with the ball into the end zone must forfeit the ball to the other team without scoring a point.
- When a goal is scored, the ball is turned over to a player on the scored-upon team, who passes it into bounds from his or her own end zone.
- The opposing team is awarded the ball — to be tossed in from the nearest sideline — when an infraction is committed; i.e. when the ball carrier holds the ball for more than five seconds, in the event of physical contact, or when a pass is incomplete. An incomplete pass is one knocked down by an opponent, caught out of bounds, or simply fumbled or missed by the intended receiver.
- Victory Ball games are completed when time expires or a certain number of points, say 15, is scored by one team.

Victory Ball Court

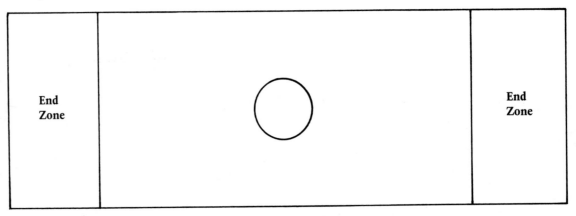

Out-of-Bounds Line

TEAM FRISBEE

With three to seven members on each team, play Team Frisbee on a rugby or football field with a goal area and marked boundaries. The object is to toss the frisbee through the opposing team's goal. Each team should have a goalie, but have players rotate so that eacfh has an equal time in goal during the game.

Team Frisbee Goal Crease

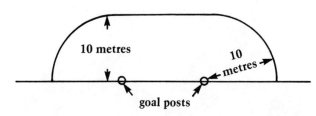

Start the game by awarding one team a free fling from centre. The following rules apply:
- Players may not walk or run with the frisbee. It is advanced by passing. It cannot be 'handed' from one player to another.
- If the frisbee touches the ground or goes out of bounds, it is to be put into play from the sideline, goal-line or in bounds point where it was dropped, by a member of the opposing team.
- If, during an attempted interception, the frisbee is touched and falls to the ground, it is to be turned over to the team opposing the last player to touch it.

- Absolutely no body contact is permitted in Team Frisbee. 'Checking' is done basketball-style. A violated player is entitled to a free fling, and players of both teams must be at least 10 m away from the flinger.
- No offensive player may enter the goal area. If this rule is violated, the defending team is awarded a free fling from inside its crease.
- If, in the opinion of the referee, a player has been prevented by illegal means (physical contact) from making what could have been a scoring shot, the offended team may select a player to take a penalty shot from any point outside the goal crease. Only the defending goalie may be in the goal area during a penalty shot.
- After a goal is scored, the scored-upon team is awarded a free fling from the centre line.

SOME VARIATIONS TO TEAM FRISBEE RULES

- Eliminate all boundaries except the goal crease.
- If the goal posts are 'H' style (for rugby), score field goals by flinging the frisbee through the uprights.
- Eliminate the need for a goal. Score by passing to a teammate in the opponent's end zone.

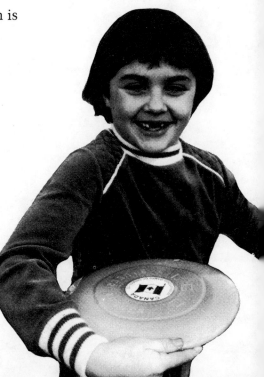

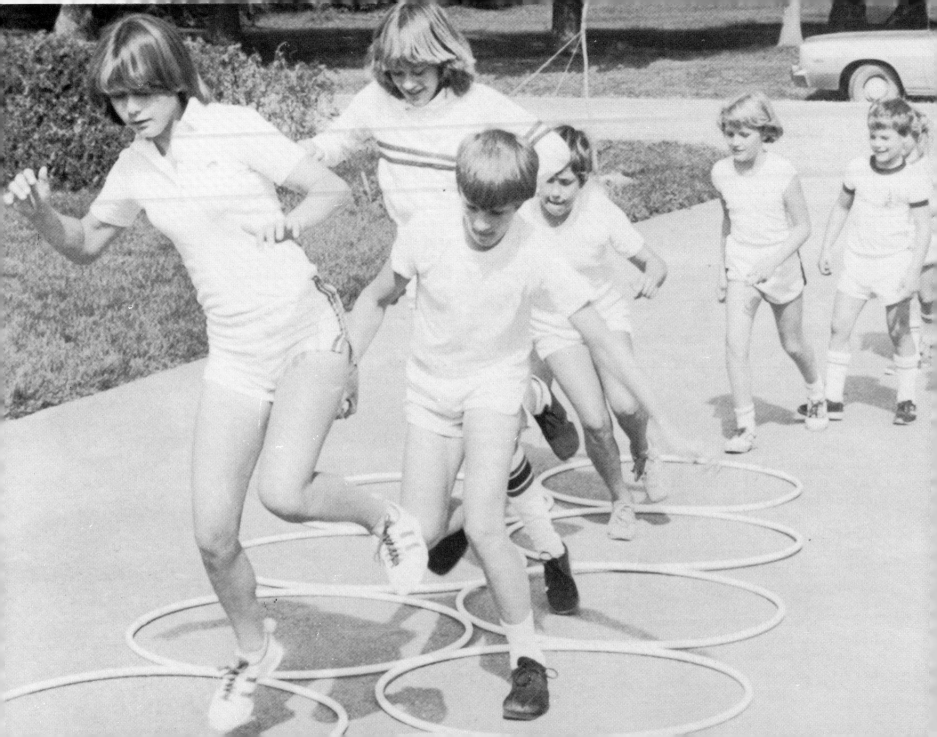

HULA HOOPS

Put down two rows of hula hoops on a flat surface or hillside. Players travel down the rows, performing one or more of the following activities, without touching any of the hoops:
- Place one foot in each hoop.
- Hop with both feet together, landing in every hoop.
- Hop on one foot only, landing inside each hoop, then hop on the other foot.
- On all fours, go straight ahead, putting one hand and foot inside each hoop.
- On all fours, go sideways.
- Run backwards, placing one foot in each hoop.

To make the Hula Hoop challenges more or less difficult, increase or decrease the spaces between the hoops.

SHORT SLALOM RUN

Place several chairs in an evenly spaced row down the length of a gymnasium. One row of chairs will serve up to ten players, but two, three or four rows can be set up for larger groups. To avoid confusion and mishap, have only one player running on each row at any one time.

Each participant starts by lying stomach down, hands next to chest, forehead on the starting line. He or she runs directly to the far wall, touches it, then returns to begin the two-way slalom of the chairs; finally, the player runs directly to the far wall once more and returns to the finish line. The instructor may wish to time the runs to see which player has the best time. Participants should be given three or four attempts to improve their times.

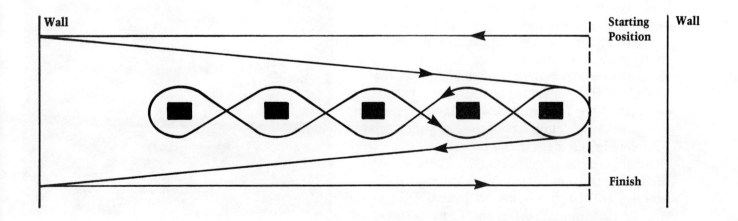

39

AEROBIC CHANCE

Post a list of six or twelve numbered excercises on a board or a large poster sheet. For example: 1. Run one lap of Gym; 2. Do ten Push-ups; 3. Do 15 Sit-ups, and so on. Adjust the exercise list to suit the environment. For instance, if the game is being played in a field include exercises like, 'Run over the bridge and around the big tree and back,' or 'Run to the four corners and back. 'Put one or two surprises in your list of exercises, such as: 2. Twiddle your thumbs for a count of 30; 3. Count someone else's Push-ups. Make certain that each player understands how to do each exercise before the game is started.

To start Aerobic Chance have each player roll one or two dice and remember the number that shows. Then start the game, with each player performing the exercise which corresponds to the number he or she threw with the dice. When all players have completed their tasks, roll the dice again. Some may roll the same exercise more than once. That's life!

Aerobic Chance can be made into a competition. If the exercises are designed to take about the same length of time to complete, then first place can be awarded to the first player to complete 10 or 15 exercises. Or, players can keep track of the numbers of the tasks they can complete in six, eight or ten minutes. If the exercises are graded according to difficulty — the higher the number, the more difficult the exercise — then the winner could be the player who first accumulates 50 points or gains the highest score in six, eight or ten minutes.

If there are more than seven in the group, have more than one set of dice so the contestants aren't forced to wait to take their toss.

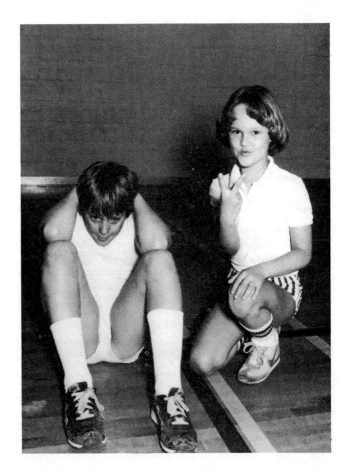

POISON PULL

Form one or more circles each of 8 to 15 players holding hands and facing inward. In the centre place hula hoop, and at a signal ask players to see if they can pull one of their number into the hoop without breaking any hand hold. When a player is dragged into or across the hoop, he or she must leave the circle to go for a short jog while the game is repeated. When a second player is pulled into the hoop and dismissed from the circle the first rejoins it, so that there is never more than one player waiting.

To end the game, allow the elimination to continue until only one player is left.

NET THE FISH

In a confined area, players form groups of four to six. One player from each group becomes a fish while the others form a linear net by holding hands. The nets chase the fish. The net must be a closed circle with the fish inside before a capture is made; a new fish is then selected. The fish cannot escape by bursting through or underneath the net.

HEAVY CATCH

This game is for two players only, one standing each side of a volleyball net or tree limb whose top is the same height as the vertical reach of the players. Each player in turn is to heave a medicine ball of manageable weight over the net to the opponent. One penalty point is scored when the ball fails to get over the net or touches the floor. A strenuous but simple game, several pairs can play over the same net at the same time. Games should only last 60 to 90 seconds because of the great effort involved.

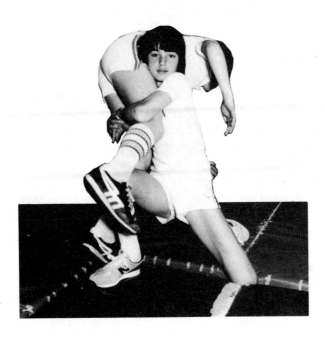

GRUESOME TWOSOMES

The following struggles are best performed by partners of equal size and strength. Instructors must discourage unnecessary roughness. Each exercise can easily be made into a round robin tournament, with players recording their own total number of victories.

One-footed Tug-of-War

Each player holds raised left foot behind the buttocks with the left hand, and partner's wrist with right hand. The player first pulled over a pre-marked line or the first to put both feet down is the loser.

Stick Lift

Players face each other, hands at shoulder width, gripping a single pole or stick. One player is to lift the stick above the level of the opponent's shoulders; the opponent is to resist with all possible might. Players may not move their feet. After a count of 20, or a succesful lift, have the players rest and reverse roles. To score, more than half the stick must be above shoulder level.

Stick Twist

In same position as for Stick Lift, except that players are permitted to move their feet, the objective of this dual is to twist the stick out of the other player's grasp. Players are not permitted to move their hands along the stick. When one hand is no longer on the stick — even for a moment — the game is won.

Cumberland Wrestle

Two players stand face to face and try to lift each other off the ground. The first to succeed wins. Neither may grab the other's clothing.

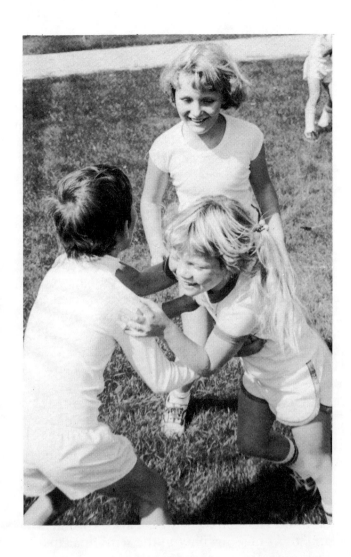

Back Down

Players sit on ground, side by side, legs straight, and facing in opposite directions. The arm closest to the opponent is to be used to try to force the opponent down on his or her back. It may not touch the opponent's head or neck. The other arm may not touch the opponent or the ground. Legs are to remain straight and together. After a victory or a count of 20, switch sides and try the same with the other arm.

Push-overs

The object of this game is to push an opponent over a line 3 m behind him or her. Push with hands on opponent's shoulders, or chest to chest with hands clasped behind back. The push must be straight: any who tries to turn an opponent is disqualified.

LIONS AND TIGERS

Two teams of equal numbers (Lions and Tigers respectively) line up facing each other, each team one giant step away from a centre line.

When the group leader shouts 'Lions', the Lions run away from the centre line towards their own safety zone and the Tigers chase them. Any Lion who is tagged before reaching the safety area becomes a Tiger for the next game. The teams line up again immediately and the group leader calls out Lions or Tigers at random, the team named being the one that must attempt to escape. The game should last six to ten minutes.

One variation is to have players start from a seated or lying position. Another variation is to call the game 'Heads and Tails' and flip a coin each round to determine which team escapes or pursues.

BULL-RINGS

The object of Bull-rings is to run after and tag one or more opponents on a circular or rectangular course.

With cones or similar objects, mark a 60-80 m track in a gymnasium or outdoors. A hillside course adds interest and effort. Single players or teams are stationed opposite and one half-lap away from their opponents.

At the starting signal, run anti-clockwise in pursuit of their opponents. An individual pursuit is ended when one player has been tagged. For team pursuits, specify in advance whether the leading, trailing or a designated runner must be tagged. The game is also ended after a specified time if no tag is made. Allow older players (15-year-olds) a longer specified time, but single runs should last no more than one minute. If a tag hasn't been made, a judge in the centre of the Bull-ring can determine which runner has gained ground on the other. Five or more individual pursuits can occur at the same time on the same track.

Organize a Bull-ring tournament to include championship and consolation rounds so that each runner has at least two runs. Seed the runners, so that fast and slow runners are paired off in the first round, with the fastest winners and losers meeting only in the semi-final and final runs. If the group doesn't have an even number of players, don't grant byes. Have two chase one, the winner advancing to the championship round and the other two to the consolation round where more doubling up will take place.

Safety Zone   Lions   Tigers   Safety Zone

44

A round robin tournament provides greater aerobic benefit because no runner has to be sidelined. Hand each runner a number. Pair off 1 and 2, 3 and 4, &c., in the first round, and keep changing the number combinations so that no runner meets the same opponent twice during the tournament. An overall winner could be declared, if necessary, on the basis of the most wins.

Bull-ring running is strenuous because it's competitive. The instructor must allow plenty of recovery time between runs, and shouldn't hesitate to withdraw from the game any runner who appears unduly fatigued.

One fun variation is **Chain Gang Bull-rings**. Form two or more teams of equal numbers of participants, who join hands with team-mates to form chains. Teams chase each other around the circle until one is tagged. If a hand hold is broken, the team must stop and link up before proceeding. A tag may not be made by a broken team, but a broken team may be tagged. Breaking up is so hard not to do!

Another Bull-ring variation, **Cut-throat Bull-ring**, is an excellent game to finish a fitness session. Place all participants equal distances apart on the Bull-ring path, all facing in the same direction. At the sound of the whistle, all run in the same direction. Any player tagged by the runner behind must drop out, until only one runner is left or a certain time, say 60 or 90 seconds, has lapsed. Not for the faint-hearted!

A number of mobility modes can be employed in Bull-rings. For example, children could pursue each other on

piggyback, making them take a 'pit stop' each lap to switch horse and rider. To confuse the issue, instruct players to reverse direction whenever the whistle is blown.

Bull-rings can be run as relays. Form teams of two or three players each, and place teams equal distances apart around the track. Have each runner run one lap qand hand a baton or bean bag to a team-mate. The game is completed when the runner of one team overtakes the runner of another. Try piggyback relays.

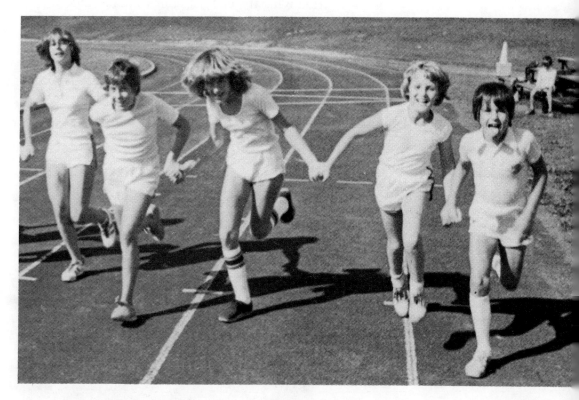

ELIMINATION HOP

Place ten bean bags or building blocks 1 m apart in a circle or straight line. Starting at any bag in the circle or at the end of a row, each participant hops on one foot over the bags, landing between each pair. After hopping over all bags, he or she bends over, without putting the other foot down, and tosses one bag aside. The player then turns and hops over the bags in the opposite direction, again eliminating the last bag. The player continues hopping back and forth and removing the end bags until none is left.

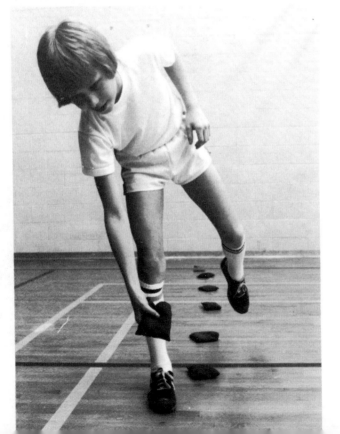

LIFT AND LAUGH

Draw a circle on the ground or chalk one on a gymnasium floor (a basketball circle may suffice); it should be large enough to contain the whole group on a standing-room-only basis.

Now explain the rules of this zany, rather rough game. Any player who is lifted off his or her feet by another must leave the circle. Safety is the first consideration. It's not necessary to lift anyone more than a few centimetres. No player can be dropped anywhere except back onto his or her feet. A player who is too aggressive, violates the simple rules, or steps out of the circle, is disqualified. One who is pushed out may return. Finally, only two will be left in the ring and everyone can bet on their favourite and laugh at the action. To make it even more aerobic, have disqualified players touch four walls of the gymnasium so they qualify to re-enter the circle. If this rule is employed, stop the game after two minutes.

Lift and Laugh can also be run as a double knockout or round-robin tournament.

FOUR WALLS

The assignment: 'Starting and finishing at any place of your own choosing, touch all four walls of the gymnasium.'

Is there a shortest route? Count to 30 while players puzzle over it, then tell them to choose their start-finish spot. The first to complete the assignment and sit down is the winner.

In the next Four Walls game, tell players to touch all four walls in succession and keep right on running until they have touched all walls (in the same order) four times. Expect some happy chaos!

Then have the players work in piggyback pairs, changing horse and rider after every second wall-touch.

MAT CLASH

Divide the group into teams of three or four players. Designate one mat for each team. Put the mats in the centre of the gym and the teams around the edge of the gym, at equal distances from their mats. The object is for each team to bring its mat to its own area of the gym; the winning team is the first to do so. Each team can try to prevent the others from retrieving their mats, but prevention methods must be non-violent. This game requires strategy, speed and strength.

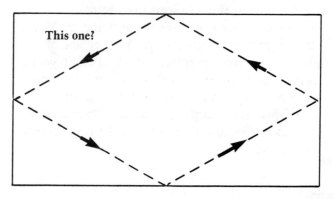

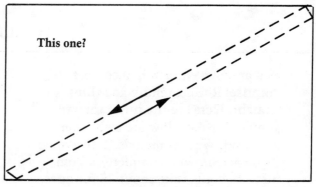

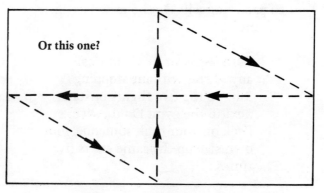

47

SURPRISE

At the start of the workout distribute a 'Surprise' list of exercises to each player. Make the aerobic exercises suit the average age of players, say five exercises for six to eight-year-olds, and up to ten for 13 to 15-year olds. For exercise ideas, turn to the sections on individual, pair and running exercises. One variation is to have the youngsters do the Surprise game list in pairs.

If you have a small group, you may have enough time to assign different numbers of repetitions for each listed exercise, based on each individual's ability.

When devising exercises, take advantage of the immediate environment. For instance, if there's a hill, have players run up it backwards.

Below is a sample Surprise game for a fit 15-year-old.

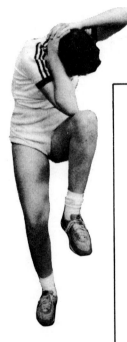

SURPRISE

You are now entered in a contest. Surprise! Read carefully and think straight. Here are the rules: they're simple. Listed below are eight exercises and two rest periods. The winner is the person who completes all ten first. It should take about 35 minutes, so pace yourself. Do the exercises in any order.

1. Run easily for five minutes, anywhere, without stopping.
2. Run up the two flights of stairs next to the gym. Do it twice.
3. Pack on your back someone your own size up the same stairs five times.
4. Rest two minutes in front of gym clock.
5. Run twice around the school.
6. Do 90 Sit-ups. (Rest as many times as you need.)
7. Sprint ten lengths of the gym, and walk — don't run — back to the start after each length.
8. Rest two minutes.
9. Do 40 standing Twisters.
10. Do 55 Push-ups. (Rest as many times as you need.)

Name _____ Total _____

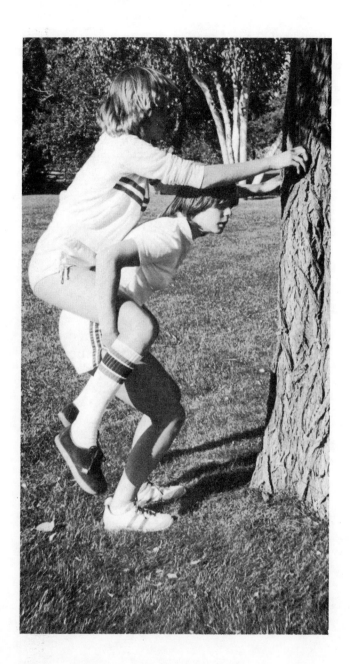

PIGGYBACK GAMES

Piggybacking is not recommended for youngsters under nine. For the following games and challenges, pair players of approximately equal size and strength.

Piggyback Race In a gymnasium or on flat ground outdoors, mark a course of 10-25 m. In the race, have pairs switch places after each length and return to the start-finish line. It is better to have frequent role-switching than to have one player bear the burden for a long distance, say 200 m.

Piggyback Relay Divide group into sets of three. Place sets at equidistant stations around a short track. Two of each set form a piggyback team and at the signal run or walk swiftly to the next station where the horse takes a rest, the rider becomes the horse, and the waiting youngster becomes the rider. The new teams then go to the next station where the process is repeated. The mounting, dismounting and galloping should go on until either all players are back at their original stations, or the relay breaks down in laughter and confusion.

Piggyback Combat This rather rough game is appealing to older players. The object is for the rider to pull another rider off his or her mount. For safety, Piggyback Combat is best played on grass or a mat. Rider and horse must switch roles often to obtain equal aerobic benefit.

Piggyback Pillow Fight Self explanatory! Take care that blows with the pillow are aimed at players' backs, not heads. Again, switch partners often.

Piggyback Polo Divide the group into two teams. Organise pairs of equal-sized players, one partner on the other's back and holding a hockey stick. The object is to bat a tennis or similar ball into the opponent's goal. The goal can be of any size and doesn't need a goal-keeper. No holding, body contact or intimidating with sticks is permitted. A penalty is 30 seconds or one minute of enforced rest on the sidelines,. Horses and riders may switch at any time, but the ball may only be struck by a mounted player. Played inside or outside, boundary measurements should be suited to the age and skill of the players. Any number may play.

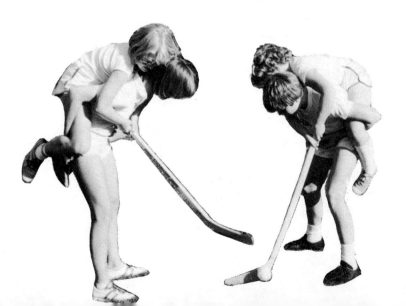

Piggyback Tag Played in the same way as regular tag, except that the pursuers and pursued are piggyback pairs. The group leader can have players reverse roles at random or on whistle signals at regular intervals.

One variation of Piggyback Tag is to play regular tag (that is, with all players on foot), until a tag is made, when the tagged player must piggyback the 'tagger' back to a designated home base. Both can then pursue others until only one untagged player is left.

In a second variation, play regular tag, but make piggyback pairs immune. That means that a pursued player may jump on the back of another for safety. Provided the other player is willing to be a horse, that is.

Piggyback Hill Race and Relay To gain even more aerobic and strength benefits, perform Piggyback Races on a hill-side. Piggyback only uphill, not down. When a pair reaches the top (or the turn-around point), they should run separately back to the start-finish line, where a new rider and horse will start off again. Or, in a short one-way race, the mid-point could be marked and the players instructed to switch roles there.

Piggyback Limbo Set up high-jump standards, the crossbar equal to the height of the tallest member of the group. Have pairs take turns going under the bar, lowering it by a few centimetres after each attempt, and eliminating the pairs who knock it off until all have failed. Switch horse and rider and play the game again.

CHAPTER 3
New Fun in Old Games

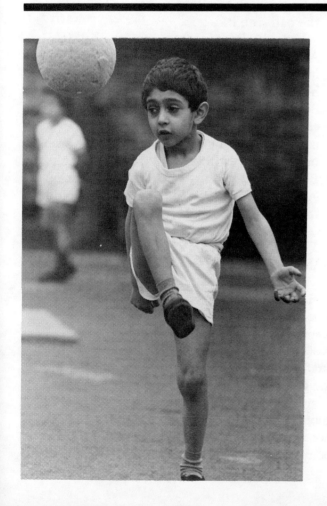

BASKETBALL FOR CHILDREN

Children usually have difficulty playing traditional basketball because the baskets are too high and some of the skills, such as dribbling, are too challenging. But basketball is one of the best aerobic games, particularly when played on a full court, and modifications can be made to make it appealing to youngsters. The following variations are suggested for their aerobic benefit and their suitability for young athletes:

- Eliminate rebounds. This means a team may only shoot once before the ball is turned over to the opponents.
- Eliminate foul shots. If a foul is committed, the fouled team automatically is awarded two points, and retains possession of the ball.
- Allow a team no more than ten seconds to take a shot.
- Have three or four players per side. (Play full-length when possible.)
- Never have players on the bench. It's better to have six or eight players on each side than to bench two or three.
- Lower the basket to 2 m.
- Use a smaller, junior model basketball.
- Where baskets aren't available, suspend old tyres or inflated inner tubes from trees or other objects. The object is to shoot the ball through the tube. For smaller players, place a hula hoop on the floor and score by bouncing the ball into it.
- When a basket is scored, keep the ball in play. Any player who gets possession of the ball as it comes through the basket can keep it for his or her team and continue play.
- Put two balls in play, and have a referee for each. Start the game with a jump ball at centre. The same players jump for the second ball and players follow the one of their choice.
- Eliminate dribbling. The ball may only be advanced by passing. No player may hold it for more than three seconds.

BASKETBRAWL

Besides scoring baskets, the object of this game is to remember which players are on which teams. Some large gymnasiums have a main basketball court, and two smaller courts at right angles to and intersecting the main one. Divide the group into six teams and play three games, using all three courts simultaneously. Expect confusion. Apply most basketball rules, but do not award foul shots: award fouled teams two points instead.

AEROBIC HOPSCOTCH

There are numerous ways to play Hopscotch. Three versions of this traditional child's game are described here. To improve the aerobic challenge, draw large squares and have one Hopscotch pattern for every two players so no-one has to wait too long for a turn.

1. Traditional Hopscotch pattern

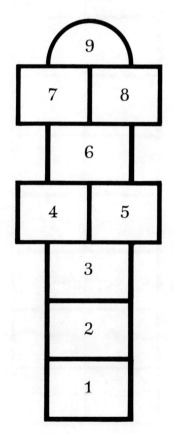

In the first two games, Traditional and Snail Hopscotch, throw a stone or small string of beads onto Square 1. Hop on one foot *over* the square containing the beads and continue hopping, touching each square, up to the highest numbered square. Turn round and hop back, hopping *over* the square with the beads. Pick up beads, toss them into the second square, and repeat the one-legged hopping. Continue until you either fail to toss the beads into the appropriate square, or step on a line while hopping. At that point, your partner takes over, and begins again at Square 1.

2. Snail pattern

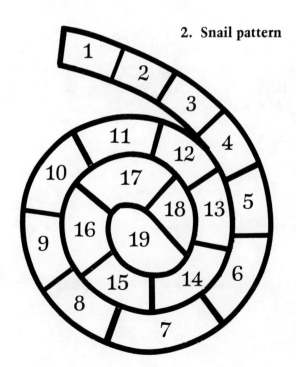

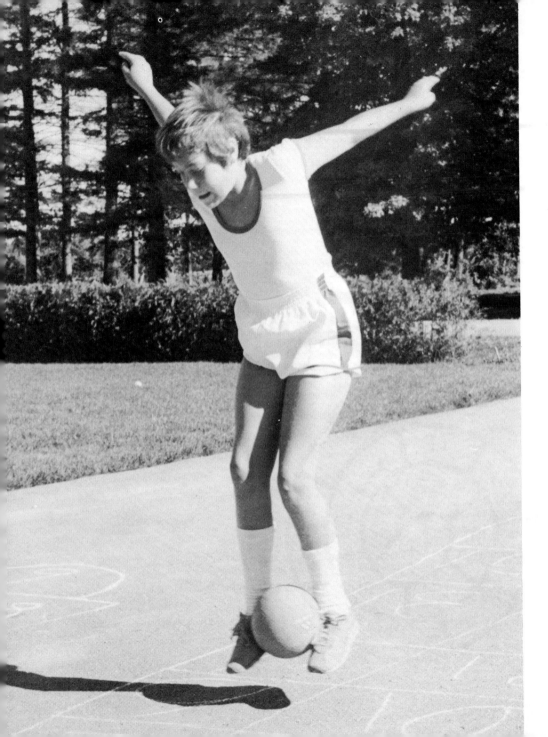

In **Two-legged Hopscotch** each player jumps through Squares 1 to 16 and back to 1 with a ball or stone gripped between his or her feet. If the ball drops, or the player steps on a line or goes into the wrong square, he or she retires and the next player begins.

1	2
3	4
5	6
7	8
9	10
11	12
13	14
15	16

HOCKEY FOR CHILDREN

Hockey, in all its forms — on ice, concrete, grass or gymnasium floor — is an excellent aerobic game for all players except the goalie. The basics are the same in all these games: the ball or puck is propelled by hand-held sticks. Sticks can be dangerous, and should not be raised above waist-level or used in any way to touch or threaten an opponent. In recent years, the wearing of face masks in minor hockey has dramatically reduced the incidence of eye injuries.

Here are some appealing hockey variations:
- Use a short-handled broom and utility ball instead of a stick and puck. Broom hockey can be played inside or outside.
- Mass Field Hockey is played outside on a soccer field. Line up each team behind its own goal-line. At a signal, the teams rush forward to a field hockey ball placed at midfield. The object is to hit the ball across the opponent's goal-line. As children improve their skills, a narrower goal can be used. After a goal is scored, line up teams as at the start of the game. No contact is permitted.

FRISBEE TENNIS

Using the scoring system and most of the rules of tennis, play singles frisbee on a normal tennis court with a net. Use the doubles court's side-lines. The end-lines are the bottoms of the back fences. Points are scored when the frisbee sails out of bounds, or when a player fails to catch it before it hits the playing surface. 'Serves' are taken from behind the regular playing serving line and must be made into the diagonal courrt, extended to the back fence. The frisbee must be returned immediately from the place it is caught. As in tennis, players serve alternate sets, but unlike tennis, each serve counts. There are no double faults or second chances.

LEAPFROG

Form a line of youngsters one behind the other, 1-2 m apart, and all facing in the same direction. They should crouch so their backs are parallel to the ground, with their hands flat on the ground near their feet for support. For safety, heads should be forward, chins tucked close to the chest.

To start, the last player in the row moves forward, leapfrogging over the players in front on the way. At the front of the line, the player crouches down again. Meanwhile, another player, finding him or herself at the back of the line, has started to leapfrog forward. This means that several players will be leapfrogging at one time. Because of the temptation to 'cheat' (by taking an extra step or two), Leapfrog isn't a good race or relay mode. But teams of two or more can have fun and good exercise leaping over each other as they go around a track, the school or a football field.

OBSTACLE COURSE

Most children love to negotiate a well-devised obstacle course. Almost anything, including the family dog, can be an obstacle, but some, such as the dog, are worse choices than others. The obstacle course can be used in a race or relay, although frantic speed may increase the chance of injury and line-ups may form at the more difficult obstacles.

A physical education equipment room will provide all sorts of appropriate obstacles. Place several chairs in a row and instruct the players to zig-zag through them, or alternately crawl under one and step over the next. Lay out mats and have players do one somersault on each mat; do a 'weiner' (or log) roll on another mat. A double row of hula hoops is a versatile obstacle. Instruct players to scale a high vaulting box, swing on ropes, high-jump a low bar into a foam rubber pit, and generally use their ingenuity to overcome impediments put in their path.

Outside, make use of sturdy fences, narrow streams, low (inexpensive!) shrubs, dust bins (for leapfrogging), and string a low rope between two trees so that players can go hand-over-hand from one tree to the other. To add difficulty, have players carry one or two medicine balls around the course.

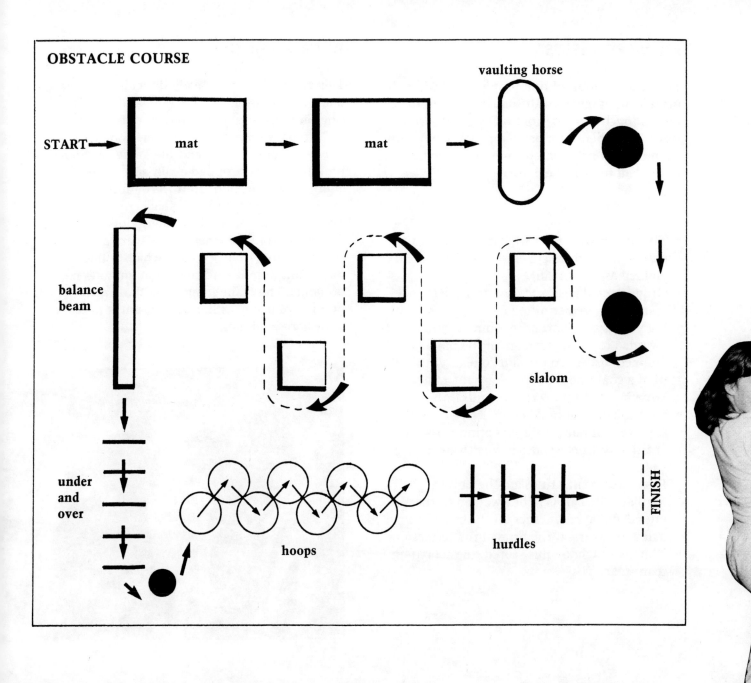

OBSTACLE COURSE

START → mat → mat → vaulting horse

balance beam

slalom

under and over

hoops

hurdles

FINISH

57

FORWARD PASSES

This is a variation of rugby, and the object is to make continuous forward passes to team-mates until a touchdown is scored. Divide group into teams, and then form pairs, a player from each team in each pair. One team is given possesion of the ball to start the game.

- The player with the ball is entitled to a free pass (i.e. not to be checked as in basketball or tackled as in football).
- Only forward passes of 4 m or more to a team-mate are permitted.
- If a pass is too short or incomplete, the ball is awarded to the other team at the point it dropped, except in the end zone or within 9 m of a goal line, in which case it can be brought out to the 9 m (10-yard) line.
- No time-outs or huddles.
- A player catching or intercepting a pass is entitled to three strides before throwing a pass.
- Pass interference rules are the same as in football: the ball is to be awarded to the offended player whether on the offensive or defensive team at the time of the infraction.
- When a touchdown is scored, the scored-on team takes possession.

BUCK PASSING

This game of catch is made difficult by the fact that those passing the ball (any kind will do) ride on their opponents' backs. Whenever the ball drops, everyone yells; whereupon all the horses become riders, and the game continues until the ball is dropped again and there is another switchround. To thwart efforts to catch the ball, horses may buck, shake, or take any disruptive action, short of falling down. The referee must judge whether a player has held the ball more than five seconds, which is the maximum time it is to remain in any one pair of hands. The team completing the largest number of passes is the winner, if it is necessary to declare a winner.

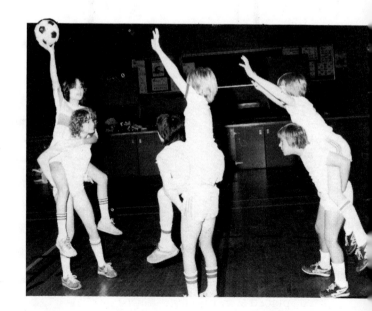

HORSEMEN OF THE APOCALYPSE

This rough and tumble affair should be conducted only on grass or large mats.

Form two teams of piggyback pairs and send them all into the fray. The object is to force the riders of the other team to touch the ground. When a pair has been grounded, it must remain out of the action until all the pairs on one team have been grounded. Then all the riders become horses and the game is repeated. The winning team is the one with the fewest grounded pairs after two rounds.

Pulling is legal, but no punching, butting, or other dirty tricks. The horse is not permitted to use hands.

One variation is to have every pair fend for itself, the winning pair being the last standing. Switch horses and riders and repeat.

SOFT LACROSSE

By eliminating body checking and expensive equipment, Lacrosse can be turned into an enjoyable aerobic game for youngsters aged between 10 and 15. There should be no more than nine youngsters per side — a goalkeeper, three defensive players, four forwards and one centre. The game is played outdoors on a field sized according to the number of players. Standard hockey or field Lacrosse goals should be used, placed 9 m inside the end-lines. Use a 20 cm diameter soft sponge ball, not a standard hard Lacrosse ball. Protective gear is optional except for the goalie, who should definitely wear a mask, body and leg pads, and gloves.

The following rules apply:
- When the ball goes out-of-bounds or penalties occur, the ball is simply turned over to the opposing team.
- On face-offs, all players except the two centres must be 5 m from the ball and may not move until the ball is released. Face-offs are held after a goal is scored, when the referee is uncertain which team last touched a ball that went out-of-bounds, and to start play.
- No player may be within 6 m of a player bringing a ball into play until that player has stepped over the sidelines.
- No player except the goalie is permitted to enter the goal crease, an arc 4 m in radius measured from the centre of the goal. No defensive player may carry the ball into his or her own crease.
- Only a goalkeeper may touch the ball with a hand.
- Stick-to-stick contact of a non-dangerous nature is permitted.
- Not more than two players from each side may scramble for a loose ball.
- Players who play dangerously may be ejected from the game.

TOUCH RUGGER

Few similarities exist between this version of Touch Rugger and the real game of rugby. There are no converts, line-outs, scrums, tackling or place-kicks. You can either use a rugby ball or a football. Choose 3 to 12 players for each side and play on a field of a size suitable to the number and age of players.

- Have one team start the game by kicking the ball from the centre line into their opponent's end.
- On any kick, if the ball is not advanced 9 m, it is turned over to the opposing team.
- The ball may be advanced by running with it or kicking it, but not by forward passes.
- The ball may be passed, under or over-handed, laterally or behind the player tossing the ball.
- When a player carrying the ball is touched by an opponent, he must kick it towards the opponent's goal.
- No player on the kicker's team may be closer than the kicker to the opponent's goal line at the moment the kick is made. Whenever an offside infraction is committed, the ball must be turned over to the opposing team at the point where the kick was taken.
- No opposing player can interfere with a kick being made as a result of a 'touch'.
- If the ball goes out of bounds, the opposing team should throw it in, either laterally or behind but not forward of the point where the ball went out.

- No body contact is permitted, except to touch a ball carrier.
- After a score is made, the 'scoring' team must kick the ball from its centre-line to its opponent's end.
- A kicked ball caught by a defending team in its own end zone does not count as a score and it may be kicked or run out.

SCORING

Try (carry over) .... 3 points
Drop Kick (through the uprights) .... 3 points
Punt (no score if ball bounces into end zone) .... 1 point
Touching a ball carrier in his or her end zone .... 1 point

SINGLES VOLLEYBALL

When it's played by senior leagues and inter-national players, volleyball is not a game with great aerobic value, but reducing the number of players to only one or two per side turns it into an aerobic game of the first order. The net must be raised, forcing the ball to go high and therefore giving each player more time to get to it. It may be necessary to reduce the court size. In the singles game, each player is permitted to bat the ball gently in the air before hitting it over the net. In doubles volleyball, a maximum of three hits is permitted per side.

Tug of War

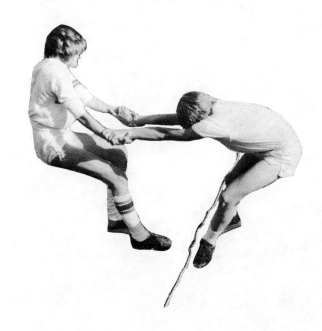

TUG OF WAR

This can be the most strenuous of games, so instructors must not allow any single 'pull' to last more than 15 seconds.

Divide the group into two teams of equal numbers and sizes, and have teams form parallel lines, facing each other and about 1 m apart. Players should alternate, so that each player is opposite a gap in the facing team. Place a strong rope between the two lines, with players grasping it at shoulder height. At a signal, each team tries to pull the other back across a line 2-3 m behind it. Stop the tug after 15 seconds. Then, from the same starting position, have players push against the rope.

In variation of this game, the teams line up, 6-12 m away from the rope and at opposite ends of a field or gymnasium. At a signal, the players rush for the rope and try to push it across the other team's end-line. No player may hold more than a shoulder's-width length of rope.

THREE MEN IN A TUG
(For three or six players)

Place a strong rope on the ground in the form of a triangle with a knot at each corner. About 2-3 m out from each knot place a bean bag or other 'prize' on the ground. Have one or a pair of youngsters lift and hold the rope at each knot with one hand (leaving the other hand to reach for the prize). At the word 'Go', each individual or pair will try to pull the opponents so the prize can be reached.

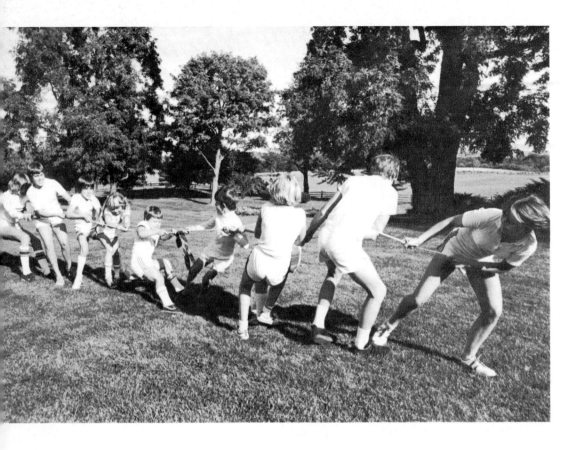

TEAM TUG OF WAR

Form two equal teams and line team members up, one behind the other, on opposite sides of a centre line. The front members of the two teams should be 3-6 m apart. The object of the game is to pull the other team across the centre line. Partial marks can be scored if one team moves the other towards, though not across, the line in the short time allotted.

To increase Tug of War fun, try this variation: line the teams up 30-60 m apart, or against opposite gymnasium walls, facing each other. On the ground equidistant from each team place a sturdy rope with a knot or ribbon at its mid-point. At the sound of the whistle, each team charges for the rope and tries to drag it, particularly the mid-point, towards its own end. There are no rules about where each individual should grab the rope — it could be either side of the mid-point — but body contact with opposing players is not permitted.

Or, try this variation of Team Tug of War. Have teams form parallel lines, facing each other across a centre line, so that each member can clasp the left wrist of one opponent in the left hand and the right wrist of another opponent in the right hand. At the sound of the whistle each team tries to pull the other across the line.

INDIVIDUAL TUG OF WAR

Two contestants stand facing each other and grasp each other's wrists in a locking grip. The game is over when one succeeds in pulling the other 5 m back from the starting point. Again, partial marks can be scored for progress.

One delightful variation is for the players to stand back to back, reach between their legs and hold hands in a non-slip grip, and then begin to tug each other.

Hold an Individual Tug of War Tournament and include a consolation round for the losers of the first matches. Because each pull is short, a Tug of War tournament for a large group can be held in just a few minutes.

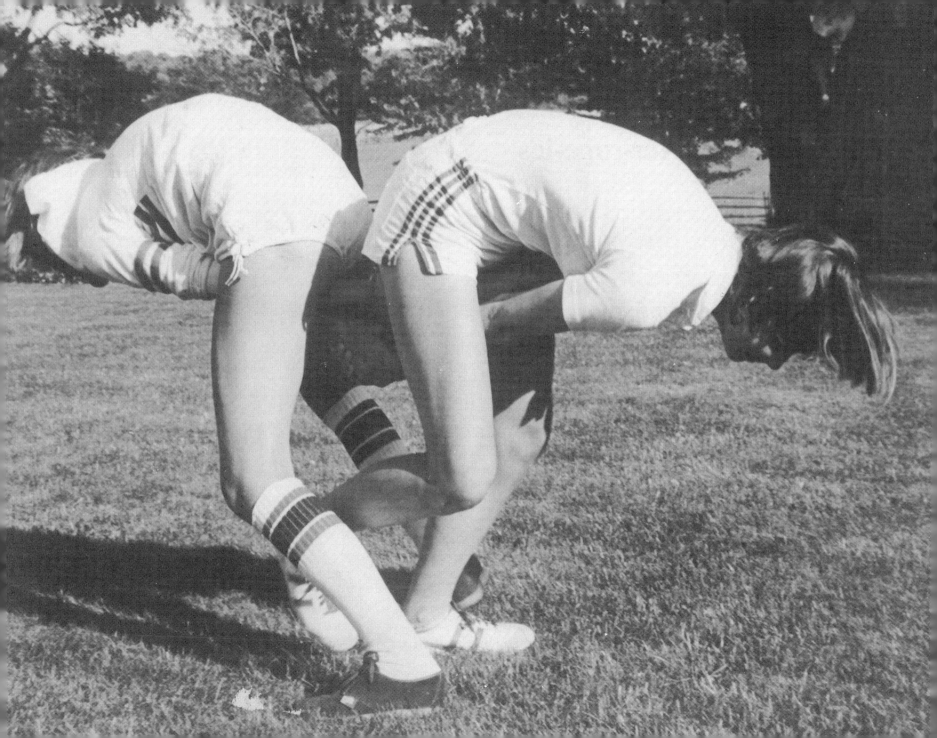

Aer-rope-ics

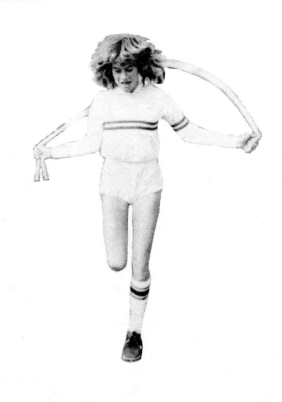

SKIPPING

No fitness program should skip skipping. Its positive effects on fitness have long been recognized by boxers and other endurance athletes. It builds leg, ankle and foot strength, coordination and timing. There are many skipping routines: on one, two or alternating feet; turning the rope backwards; taking two jumps per rope turn; running or jumping forwards on two feet while skipping; or using a short rope, (which calls for very strenuous high leaps).

To obtain proper rope length, stand on the approximate centre of the rope, spread feet comfortably apart, and pull the rope ends up to the waist. If there is extra rope, tie knots at waist level to show where it should be held.

Begin skipping by holding elbows and shoulders steady and moving forearms, wrists, and hands. Keep arms close to sides. Land lightly on the front (balls) of the feet, and keep knees slightly flexed. Look ahead, not down. To increase the aerobic benefit of skipping, increase the frequency of jumps or jump higher.

Do the following routines for 30 seconds each. Some may be too advanced for young or inexperienced skippers. They should keep practising the simple exercises while others are doing the difficult ones.

- Skip on both feet, swinging rope forwards.
- Skip on both feet, swinging the rope backwards.
- Skip on both feet, taking two bounces with each full turn of the rope.
- Skip around the gym.
- Skip on right foot.
- Skip on left foot.
- Alternate left and right feet, touching one foot down with each rotation.
- Cross arms with each rotation.
- High-leg-lift skipping, with shortened rope.
- Using short rope, pass it under one leg at a time with each walking step around an indoor track.

SKIPPING GAMES FOR PAIRS AND GROUPS

Double Jump One player turns a long rope while standing toe-to-toe or toe-to-heel with a partner. Skip for 30 to 45 seconds, then allow partner to turn the rope for another 30 to 45 seconds.

Circle Skip Line up players equal distances apart in a circle. The player in the middle whirls a weighted rope longer than circle's radius. Other players must jump over it. Starting just above ground level, the rope may not be brought up higher than mid-shin. Any player who touches the rope must tag all four walls, or (if outside) run to a designated point and back, before being allowed back into the circle. The player in the middle must be changed often to prevent dizziness.

A Ropeless Cause Divide group into two teams. Every member of one team takes a skipping rope and holds it lightly between the thumb and fingers. They then run around the gym, dragging and wiggling the ropes behind them. Members of the ropeless team must chase them, and try to stamp on a rope. Anyone who succeeds in stamping on a rope takes possession of it, and the game continues.

Skipping Races Use either a normal sprinting action while turning the rope, or jump forwards with two feet together turning the rope once with each skip.

Skipping Relays Using either the sprinting or jumping style, form teams of two or three for relays around a short running loop.

Under the Moon Two players turn a rope for a third player who jumps in and skips once, then jumps out; then jumps in again for two skips, and so on, up to ten. Change roles often so that each player has plenty of skipping time.

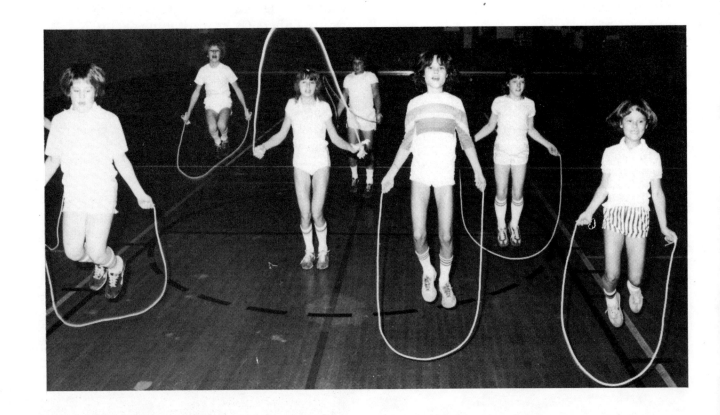

ROPEY ROUTINES
(Use a 3-5 m rope if possible)

Rope Climbing Shimmy up and down a firmly anchored rope, using arms and legs. Or, climb up and down rope without using legs. (For older, stronger participants.)

- Place rope on floor in straight line. Jump on both feet back and forth across it ten times.
- Turn in the air and land facing the opposite direction with each jump, ten times.
- Repeat these exercises first on right foot, then on left.
- On one foot zig-zag length of rope, turn and return. Repeat on other foot.
- Zig-zag length of rope alternately putting down hands together and feet together. That means feet will remain on one side of the rope, hands on the other.
- In push-up position, hands on one side of rope, feet on the other, walk sideways for length of rope, and return. Turn over, and repeat exercise in crab-walk position.
- Repeat the last exercise, but keep right foot off the floor at all times, then left foot.
- Shape the rope as a triangle and jump on both feet across it, so that feet land together outside each side of the triangle. Jump around the triangle three times, then do the same on one foot, then the other.

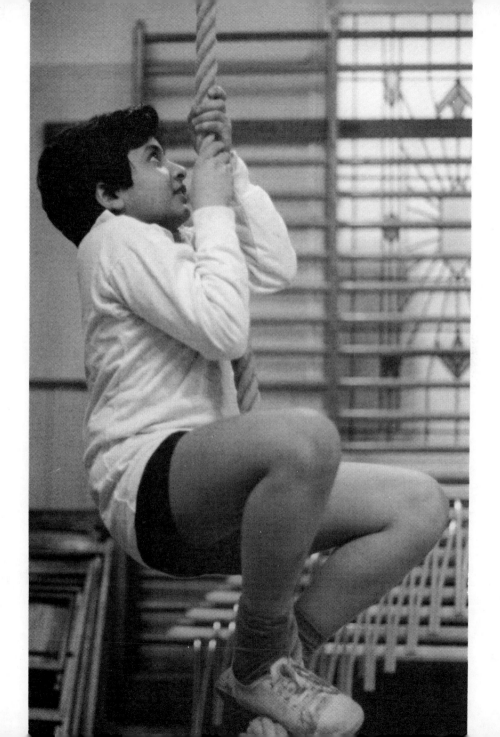

Soccer for Children

SOCCER

The origins of soccer, the world's most popular team sport, go back at least as far as 14th-century Britain. Soccer then was truly an aerobic contest, with goals often set kilometres apart, and the playing area containing such obstructions as streams, woods, farm animals, hills and valleys. Primitive soccer is not a bad idea for an instructor looking for a 'different' sort of sporting adventure. Try a game of 'Medieval Football' in a large farm field (after the crops have been harvested) or other open area. Suit the rules to the landscape and the number of players.

More civilized rules were not added to soccer until the 19th century, and it is unfortunate that so many minor sports organizations seem compelled to impose the rules so strictly.

Soccer is an ideal aerobic game for youngsters. Like a swarm of bees, six- to ten-year-olds will follow the ball wherever it goes. Remembering that fitness and fun are the first objectives, instructors should not spend half the activity hour teaching the virtues of positional play, particularly if it means that more obedient youngsters will cover their zones diligently and never get a chance to kick the ball. Later, as their skills improve, help players learn that passing and positional play will bring goals.

Whenever possible, put all youngsters on the field. If it is necessary to have a goalie — it's a sedentary life in goal — rotate the position so that no-one stays in goal too long. For indoor games, let some air out of the ball so it cannot be kicked too hard.

Soccer provides a valuable opportunity for continuous running. It is simple to understand and can be played with equal joy by boys and girls of all ages and skill levels. Games and leagues are relatively easy to organize.

MINI SOCCER

A mini-soccer programme recently organised for youngsters under ten has been highly successful. The mini-soccer leagues have reduced the number of players on teams and use a lighter ball and smaller field and goal. These changes increase each player's time with the coach and contact with the ball, which can be more easily headed, kicked, trapped, dribbled and thrown. Having fewer than the regular 11 players decreases the tendency to bunch up and encourages team work.

- Mark two small fields side by side on a standard soccer field. Small fields are better suited to the size, strength, perspective and ability of the players.
- For players under eight, a portable goal 1.5 m high can be constructed from pipes so that the crossbar can telescope, allowing goal widths of 2.5 - 3.5 m.
- Divide the game-time into 10 or 12 minute quarters with a short break in between. To reduce penalties and interruptions, eliminate the offside rule, do not allow the goalkeeper to hold the ball outside the goal crease (an arc with a 5 m radius from the centre of the goal), and do not permit intentional body contact.
- For a goal to count, the ball must be shot from outside the goal arc. Defenders may stand inside the goal area, and a ball that deflects off a defending player(s) into the goal may be counted. Penalty shots should be taken from a spot 9 m directly in front of the goal.
- One coach or parent for each team may be on the field during play, but should not interfere with play in any way. No adults are allowed in the goal area or behind the goals.

Recommended Field Dimensions						
Age	Playing Field		Goal		Ball	
	Length	Width	Width	Height	Circ.	Size
8-10	73 m	44 m	5 m	1.8 m	55 cm (approx.)	2
10-12	77 m	45 m	5 m	1.8 m	60 cm (approx.)	3
12-14	91 m	53 m	6 m	2 m	65 cm (approx.)	4
14-16	95 m	60 m	7 m	2.5 m	70 cm (approx.)	5

ONE-PASS SOCCER

Regular soccer, except that no player is permitted to dribble the ball. He or she may only kick it once before another player touches it. This rule forces youngsters to pass the ball and practise teamwork. A point is awarded to the opponents if a player touches the ball twice or more in succession. Scoring a goal counts five points.

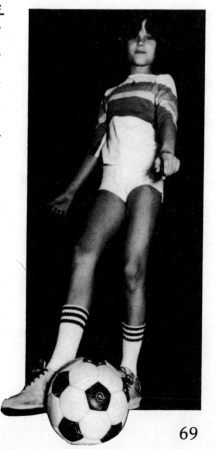

HAND SOCCER

Indoor Hand Soccer is an exciting, fast-moving aerobic game. The ball — a deflated soccer ball, basketball, volleyball or large utility ball — may only be struck with one hand, not two hands together nor feet, and it may not be carried. The end walls of a gymnasium are suitable goals; there are no goalkeepers because they don't get much exercise. The side walls are the boundary lines, so there are no throw-ins.

Choose two teams of 6 to 15 players and award one side the 'kick-off' at the centre line. Future 'kick-offs' are to be taken by the team that has just been scored against. Other rules of soccer apply.

Here's a variation of Indoor Hand Soccer. Line up each team (six to ten players) along a base line in front of its goal (end wall), and have the players link elbows. The referee then blows his whistle to signal the players from the right end of each row to come to the centre to play the game, rules as for Hand Soccer. After 30 or 60 seconds of play the whistle is blown and the players return to the left ends of their rows, while the next two from the right ends continue the game. The two rows may try to prevent a goal from being scored by using their bodies or feet, but may not unlink arms. If the arms should become unlinked a goal is automatically awarded.

If it's found that the normal game of Hand Soccer results in too many goals, and therefore too many interruptions, place an Indian Club in the centre of each of the two basketball foul-shot circles and declare the circles out-of-bounds areas for both teams. When the ball knocks over a club, it counts as a scored goal.

No body contact is permitted. Instructors must discourage youngsters from charging the ball, which is a dangerous practice because players' heads are down.

To improve participation, allow each player only one hit at a time. If a player hits the ball twice or more in succession, award a free hit to the opposing team.

CRAB SOCCER

Indoors, have players on both teams assume the crab-walk position (back down, hands and feet on the floor). It's permissible to let the seat of the pants rest on the floor and even to slide along. Players should wear gloves if possible. Most soccer rules apply; except that the end walls are goals (no goalkeepers) and the side walls are the side boundaries (no throw-ins). With more than five players per team, try putting two balls in play. Game times should be short, say four to six minutes per half, because crab walking is strenuous.

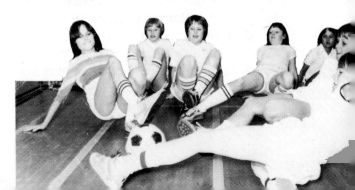

Tag

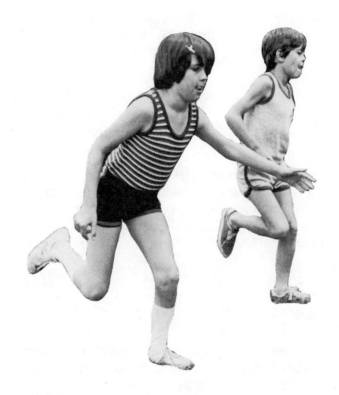

This oldest of games combines the best of aerobic running (change of pace and direction) with the best elements of a chase (surprise, excitement and anticipation). Variations are endless; some especially aerobic versions are suggested here. Mark well-defined boundaries around an area suitable in size to the number and age of the players. A small area will encourage more running and tagging, and thus provide more exercise.

BALL TAG

IT tries to throw a soft ball, such as a slightly deflated volleyball, so that it touches another player below the waist. The struck player becomes IT. This game is best played indoors where long delays — caused by retrieving the ball — can be avoided. The game may be played (even outdoors) with two ITs working together. The player hit by the ball replaces the IT who threw it.

One variation is to kick the ball instead of throwing it by hand. For this Ball Tag game, at least two ITs should work together.

HANG TAG

Played like regular Tag except that players are immune from being tagged when they are hanging from ropes or other apparatus in the gymnasium. Of course, they cannot stay up there forever. IT surely will know that and be waiting.

LINE TAG

The same rules apply as in regular Tag, except that players must run along lines on the gym floor. Anyone who steps off a line automatically becomes IT. The group leader may wish to instruct players to use lines of a certain colour.

AEROBIC IMMUNITY TAG

A pursued player may not be tagged while doing ten repetitions of Push-ups, Sit-ups, Half Squats or other aerobic exercises. IT may not hover over an exercising player, but must count to three after the pursued player's last repetition before chasing. If three exercises, say Push-ups, Sit-ups and Half Squats, are declared immunity exercises, the pursued player may only do each of these once to remain immune. For easy administration and to avoid arguments, start by declaring only one exercise valid for immunity with each new IT.

POLO TAG

Choose two teams equal in number, one team to be ITs. Each IT is given one utility ball which must remain on the floor throughout the game. The object of Polo Tag is to strike a non-IT player on the foot or lower leg with the ball. Tagged players must remove themselves to a designated area to perform one or two exercises, such as ten sit-ups, before returning to the game, again as a non-IT. An IT player may only strike the ball with a fist and may not kick the ball. At the end of each minute the group leader signals the sides to reverse roles, the IT players to become non-ITs, and vice versa.

Polo Tag can be played by almost any number of youngsters in a gymnasium. (It's difficult to control the balls on a playfield.) With unlimited boundaries indoors, most non-IT players will be able to escape being tagged, so they should be confined to a smaller square, marked by cones, covering approximately one half of the total gymnasium area. If the non-ITs run outside the square they will suffer the same consequences as if they had been tagged by the ball. ITs on the other hand need not be restricted to this central square.

SNOW TAG

Deep or new-fallen snow, dry sand and high grass provide ideal resistance for increasing aerobic and muscular effort in many games.

Games of tag using marked pathways, such as Snow Tag, can be played on almost any surface, but snow is ideal. The diagram accompanying this description is for Snow Tag with four to six players, but it's easy to create more elaborate mazes for larger numbers.

The object of the game — for everyone but the player(s) who is IT — is to avoid being tagged while remaining within the narrow channels. The metre-wide pathways can be made by trampling unmarked snow or sand, or cones on harder surfaces.

Snow Tag Maze

15 metres

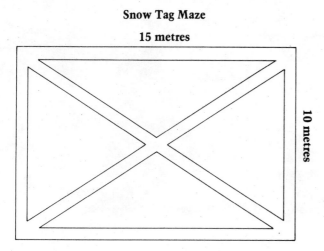

10 metres

TEAM TAG

Divide the group into two teams of equal numbers and give each team a name. Have members of one team wear bibs, hats or in some way distinguish themselves. When the group leader calls out the name of one team, that team must pursue the other. When a player is tagged, he or she must sit down. The game ends when all members of one team are sitting. The team that remains untagged for the longest time is the winner.

WATER TAG

Play regular Tag in a pool or defined area of pond, lake or ocean. Any swimmer who leaves the water to avoid being tagged automatically becomes IT.

One variation for accomplished swimmers is to have IT yell out a style of swimming (freestyle, backstroke, breaststroke, or butterfly). Any swimmer failing to use the proper stroke becomes IT.

A tag can be a direct touch or a strike by a slightly deflated volleyball tossed by IT.

OPTIONAL TAG

Divide the room or play area into halves and select one fast-running IT for each side. An IT may not go out of his or her territory, but the pursued can cross the boundary freely according to how they think they will fare in either half.

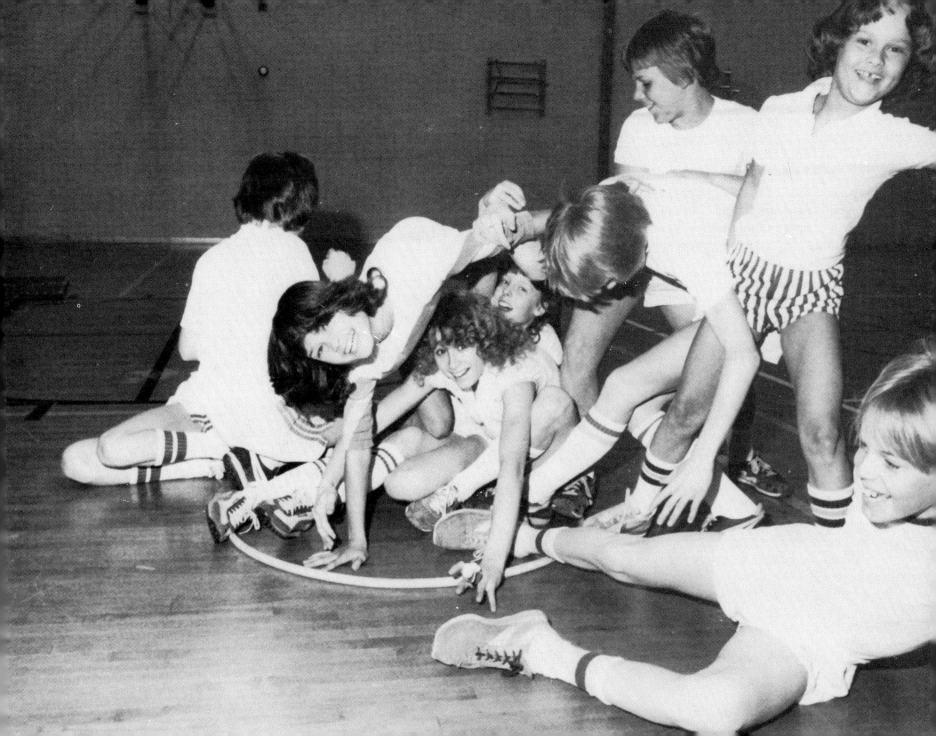

BEAN BAG TAG

Use one hula hoop for every six youngsters in the group. Place the hoops (or draw circles on the ground) close together at one end of the play area. Give one bean bag each to less than half the youngsters and assemble the remaining players in an area far away from the hoops or circles. The object of the game for non-IT players is to reach the safety of the circles. A tagged player must accept the bean bag and pursue those without a bean bag. Players who reach the circle stay there until the game is completed. To prevent too much idleness, one game should last no more than two minutes or until all players have reached hoops, whichever occurs first. ITs for the next game should be chosen from among players in the circles. Others should return to the far end of the play area before the next game is started.

DOUBLE AGENT TAG

Players who think they are gaining may be losing. Number One player chase Two, who chases Three, who chases Four, who chases One. When a tag is made, the game is over and each player is assigned a new number, so each will be chasing and avoiding a different runner. The intrigue and confusion with more than four players is always very stimulating.

ALWAYS IT TAG

Once a player has been tagged, he or she remains IT for the rest of the game. The number of IT players will increase rapidly after the initial stages of the game. The last player to be tagged is the first IT for the next game. IT players should put one hand on top of their heads to indicate they have been tagged.

CHAIN-GANG TAG

In a confined space with clearly marked boundaries, one player in every six to eight is appointed to be an IT. A tagged player joins hands with IT, and together they run to tag other players. With each tag, the chain gets longer. Only the two end players in the chain can make a tag. When there are no non-ITs left, the team with the longest chain is the winner. If the chain breaks during a chase it cannot make a tag until the break has been mended. Players should be told to shout the name of an intended victim so the chain-gang can coordinate the pursuit.

FIVE POINTS DOWN TAG

A player is immune from being tagged as long as his or her feet, hands and forehead are on the floor simultaneously. Knees may not be touched down.

COMPANION TAG

Divide the group into pairs. In a confined space, declare either the first or second partner IT. When one partner tags the other, the new IT must count to four before chasing the other partner. After one minute, have a short rest period during which new partnerships can be formed, matching players of equal ability.

CUDDLE TAG

For six to eight-year-olds (or people of any age who feel free and friendly), the regular rules of Tag apply except that players are immune from being tagged if they are cuddling (wrapping their arms around) another player. As the game progresses, declare only groups of three cuddlers immune. Then four, five, and more, until the whole group is cuddling, and then allow the lonely IT to join in.

BEE STING TAG

Appoint two to five bees (ITs). Other players are bears. Play the game inside four cones which mark the boundaries of the forest. When bears are stung (tagged) they leave the forst and walk or run around until all the other bears have been stung. The last to be stung are bees for the next game.

THREE'S A CROWD TAG

For an odd number of players, one is declared IT and the others form pairs holding hands. When IT tags a player, that player becomes IT and the former IT becomes the new partner. The new partnership is immune for as long as the former partner remains IT.

TANDEM TAG

Form pairs, linking elbows or hands, and declare one couple IT. The IT pair chases other pairs.

REVERSED PARTNER TAG

Have each pair, including the couple who are IT, link arms at the elbows while facing in opposite directions. One partner will run forwards, the other, backwards. Then follow regular Tag rules.

SHADOW TAG

IT must try to tag other players' shadows. Not recommended for dimly lit gymnasiums, cloudy days, moonless nights, or total eclipses of the sun.

POSSE TAG

A runner is given a five-second head start on an open field. The posse follows until the pursued is tagged. A short rest is taken before another runner is named and the game starts again. Never give the fastest or most enduring runner the chore of being pursued, or the game will never be concluded.

FROZEN TAG

A player freezes in the pose he or she is in at the moment of being tagged. The frozen player is released only if a non-IT player is able to crawl between his or her legs. Ratio of IT to non-IT players should be one to five. Have six periods in the game. Each period ends when all players are frozen, or after two minutes have elapsed, whichever occurs first. Have a new IT player for each period.

IMITATION TAG

Have the pursued imitate the pursuer exactly . . . run, hop, skip, crawl on all fours, make a crazy face, hold arms above head, flap arms as if to take flight, anything! If the referee sees a player failing to imitate, or making a feeble effort to imitate that player is declared IT. IT is entitled to change his or her mode of pursuit at anytime.

FLAMINGO TAG

Similar to regular Tag, with one player as IT, other players can render themselves safe from being tagged by standing on one foot and raising the knee to the other leg to hip height. Flamingoes who lose balance (without being pushed by IT) and touch both feet down, can be tagged.

A related game is **Skunk Tag**. Pursued players are safe while they hold their noses, but there's a catch; they must stand on one leg, and reach for their noses by the hand of the arm held under the raised leg.

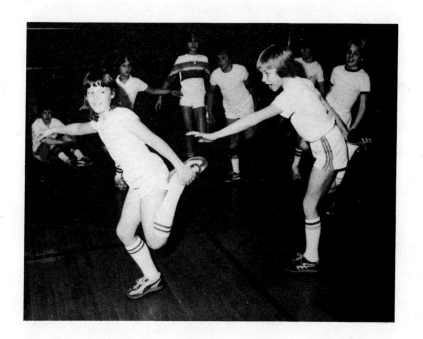

CHAPTER 4

Aerobic Races and Relays

When we think of races, we usually think of running. But races can be varied endlessly by using different movement modes. The following suggestions provide an aerobic challenge, and will entertain spectators as much as participants.

Relays involve teams, rather than individuals. They can be run competitively, as races, but need not be. The relays described later in this chapter call for a real team effort. In a simpler form, relays can use any of the movements suggested here, with each team member completing one section of the course independently.

Races

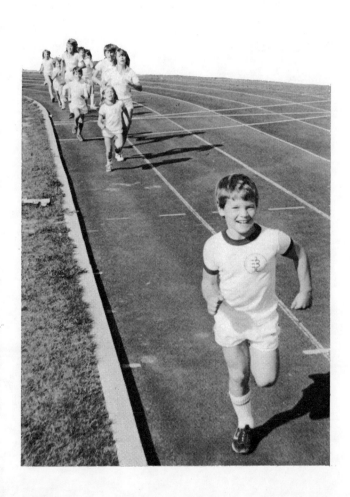

SPRINT

Very straightforward. Sprint one section of a track, or round a turning point and back.

BEAR WALK

On all fours, stomach facing down, move forwards, backwards or sideways. Pretend the bear has sore paw—perhaps it was stung by a bee and can't put down its right foot. Or challenge the bears to a co-ordination test: have them move right foot and arm at the same time, then left foot and arm, and so on.

CRAB WALK

Move on all fours, stomach up.

BOTH ARMS, ONE LEG

A challenging variation of crab and bear walks: keep one foot off the ground and move in the direction the knee is pointing.

This is a difficult and fatiguing exercise for older children only, and the race distance should be short.

BUNNY HOP

Place arms between knees, and touch hands to the floor with each hop.

CROOKED WALKING

Take a long step with the right foot, then cross the left foot behind the right foot. Then, cross the right foot behind the left foot and take a long step with the left foot. Carry on as if nobody is looking. This can be used in a race or relay, or just as a means of getting to and from school.

GAWKY RUN

Bend down and grasp left heel in left hand and right heel in right hand. Move as fast as possible without losing grip on heels.

HOP-ALONG

Hopping forwards and backwards on one or two feet is excellent for individual races or relays, building aerobic and leg strength, balance and agility. Youngsters may have difficulty with two-legged hops.

SEAL SLIDE

Assume push-up position, with toes pointed away from body (so tops of feet are resting on the floor), and move forward using only hands, letting feet slide. To save hands, this routine should be done inside or on grass over short distances. For competitive seal sliding, closely scrutinize to ensure that contestants do not gain advantage from their legs.

WORM

Lie flat on a floor, elbows down and hands near the ears. Using elbows together or alternately, pull body along the floor, with as little body movement as possible. Instruct players to keep stomach and thighs on the floor at all times.

ELEPHANT WALK

On all fours, keep legs straight.

STICKY FOOT

Carry a relay baton or bean bag between feet, crabwalk or seal slide style. If the object falls out, the player must replace it before continuing. No progress is permitted empty-footed.

RIGID LEGS

Keep legs absolutely straight while running or walking.

PARTNER HOPS

With one arm, each partner holds the other around the back of the waist. The other hand holds the ankle of the raised outside leg. Start hopping. In a relay for three-member teams, one of the first partners can become the partner of the third member for the second length.

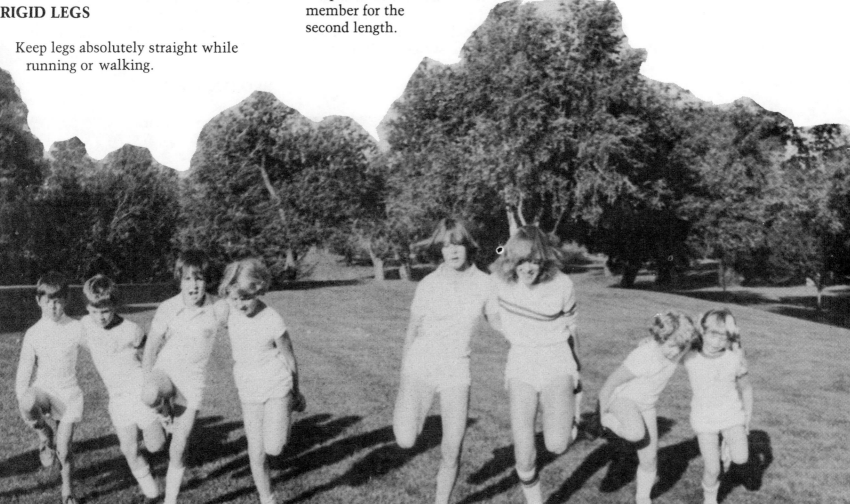

BUMS RUSH

Form chains of not more than 8 youngsters each, seated, each player with legs wrapped around the stomach of the person in front. The chains can move either feet first or backs first. Movement is made by vigorously pushing hands against the ground. Set the race distance of 6-20 m, the longer course for the older or fitter players. If, during the race, there's a split in the chain, the team must stop and re-unite before continuing.

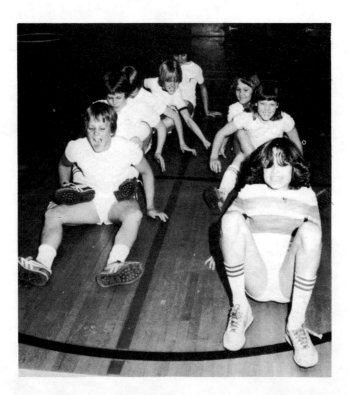

The Bums Rush should be done on a soft or smooth surface. It's not an activity to be performed while wearing one's best clothes.

Expect mild complaining and much laughter.

BACKWARDS HOP

Hop backwards on one or both feet.

BROKEN FOOT

Hold one toe or foot.

HEAVY, MAN, REAL HEAVY

Have players run races and relays holding a medicine ball or other suitable heavy object.

DEVIL TAKE THE HINDMOST

This traditional running race has considerable aerobic advantages besides being an entertainment for both instructor and participants.

Using cones, mark a circular 60 m lap indoors. Tell the group, at the starting line, to run at an easy pace for four laps; at the end of the fifth lap the hindmost runner will be removed from the race. For each of the following laps the last runner to cross the line will have to drop out. If there's a tie for last place allow both runners to remain in the race but let the entire group know that two runners will be eliminated at the end of the next lap. The race is ended when only one runner is left.

To prevent confusion don't allow the front runner to lap the last runner!

SPRINT STARTS

Children of all ages enjoy sprint starts. This programme is easily adapted to groups of all sizes; one instructor can manage a session for up to 40 youngsters.

Start with sprinter's warm-up exercises: Lean a Little, Leg Exchanges, and Sit-ups. Next, do some light jogging and four to six wind sprints of 20-60 m. Divide the group into flights of three to eight sprinters, grouping runners of equal ability. Indoors, they can place one foot against a wall; outdoors, use starting blocks and mark a finish line 15-40 m away.

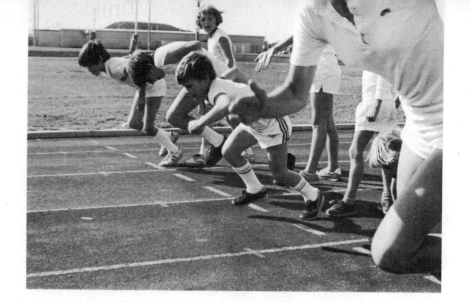

Bring the first group to the starting line and give the commands: "Runners to your marks . . . Set . . . Go!" (Blasting a starting gun will add authenticity to the effort). While the first group is sprinting, the second group moves to the start. Continue to have flights sprint in rotation.

Each youngster should run six to ten times. If the interval between races is short, each participant will have an exciting aerobic workout. The short interval is as important for the workout as the sprint itself, so don't allow time for adjusting blocks or unravelling a dispute over who won a photo-finish.

One excellent variation is to sprint uphill. This workout can also be conducted as a round-robin tournament, the fastest sprinters meeting in the final race.

SIDEWAYS SKIP

The Sideways Skip can be an individual race, a mobility mode for a relay, or simply a good aerobic exercise.

Place the outside of one foot on the floor at the base of a wall, with the body at a 90 degree angle to the wall. Skip sideways to the opposite wall and return. Turn so that the other foot is snug against the base of the wall and body is facing in the opposite direction from the first skip, then skip to the other wall and back.

When skipping, the trailing leg must never cross ahead of the lead leg. The desire to cheat on the technique is likely to increase if skippers are involved in a race or relay.

An excellent variation of the Sideways Skip is to turn 180 degrees every 1, 2, or 3 sideways strides while travelling in the same direction. If the half-turns are continued in the same direction, say to the left, then players may get dizzy. While this is fun for a short distance, it may be better to make the half-turns in alternating directions.

DRIBBLING

Bounce a basketball, dribble a soccer ball with the feet, push a volleyball along in a pool, stick handle a hockey puck, or control a ball with a broom or floor hockey stick. All these movement modes are suitable for relays or races. For relays, have each youngster dribble both directions. This will force him or her to control the ball or puck at the turn-around point.

One relay variation is to dribble one length, turn, pass the object back to the next player, and return to the end of the line, avoiding the dribbling player approaching in the opposite direction.

Another variation is to dribble around obstacles on a circular course.

BASKETBALL SHOOTING RACE

This race is appropriate for youngsters 11 and over in a gymnasium with four or six baskets. Station one or two youngsters, each with a basketball, under each basket, then dribble to the next hoop, continuing around the gym and scoring once at each basket. Score as many baskets or complete as many circuits as possible in a specified time. All players move in the same direction. No player may move to the next basket until he or she scores. For relays with two players per team, have each member go around the gymnasium once then hand the ball off to his or her partner; continue the relay for two to four minutes.

Relays

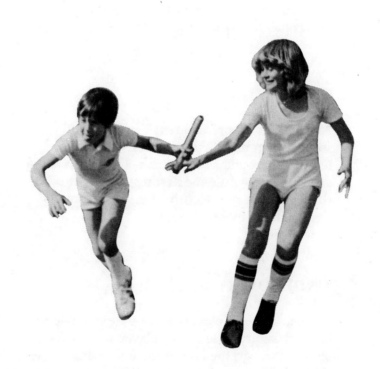

- There are two basic types of relay; shuttle (back and forth over the same bit of ground) and circuit (around a track of any size.) Run circuit relays whenever possible. This minimizes the temptation to cheat by setting off before the baton has changed hands.
- In shuttle relays, have participants run around cones placed at each end of the course: each participant runs the length of the course, rounds a cone, runs back to the start-line and rounds another cone before handing the baton over to the next runner.
- Exchange batons, beanbags, sticks or balls between each leg of a relay. This is much less confusing than relying on handslaps to indicate an exchange.
- Increase aerobic value by restricting the number of participants to three or four per team, to cut down on idle time.

STICK-WITH-IT RELAY

Have two players stand back to back holding a pole or hockey stick between their legs. The pair runs one length and then, without turning around, races back to the starting line.
The second member of the team joins the third in similar fashion. Continue the relay until each player has had two turns.

HOLDING HANDS

Form teams of three runners. The first and second team members join hands and run a length, or around a short track. Then the second and third run while the first rests. Next the third and first run. Continue until all runners have run one to four lengths.

UNDER-OVER RELAY

A team of three players assembles in single file behind a starting line. The player at the back crawls through the legs of the one in front, leap frogs the next, and then runs the length of the course, rounds a cone and returns to stand at the front of the line behind the starting line. The player now at the back of the line follows the same routine. When the players find themselves in their original positions once again, they should repeat the relay twice.

A RELAY POTPOURRI

Post a list of two to eight different movement modes near the start line of a shuttle or lap relay. Demonstrate each mode before the relay starts. After each participant has completed the first mode, he or she performs the second, then third, and so on.

THREE-LEGGED GAMES

Besides running races and relays, three-legged pairs can have fun playing a number of aerobic games, such as touch rugger, soccer, basketball and numerous games of tag. Using soft cloth or ties, strap ankles together. Join children of equal size and outlook on life.

A group of three players can form a four-legged thing.

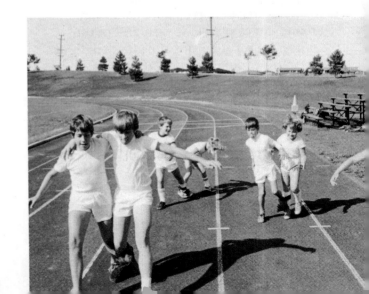

CONSTRUCTION RELAY

For six- to eight-year-olds, divide the group into teams of three. Give each player a building block. The first runner in each team runs the length of the gym or field, places his or her block on the ground, and returns to the start. The second runner then races to put another block on top of the first, and returns to the start. The third runner puts the final block on top. When he or she returns, the demolition process begins. The first team member retrieves the top block, and so on.

One variation is to provide each team with a large number of blocks and instruct them to build a tall building, using the relay format outlined. The team completing highest tower is the best team of engineers.

ADD AND SUBTRACT RELAY

The first player on a three- or four-member team runs around a short indoor or outdoor track, or runs two lengths (down and back) of a gym. On returning, the first and second join hands and run the same route, then pick up the third member, and finally the fourth. After all runners, hand-in-hand, have completed the course together, the first runner is dropped, and so on, until all have returned to the starting line.

STICK HOP RELAY

Teams of three form lines behind a start line. In front of each team, at the other end of the course, a pole or metre stick is placed on the ground.

The first runner in each team races to the metre stick, picks it up, and returns to the start-line. Holding the stick at knee height, he or she runs past the other members of the team who must jump over the stick. The runner races around the last team member holding the stick at waist height. As he or she returns, other team members must duck under it. The runner then races to deposit the stick at the other end of the course, and returns to the back of the line. The second member of the team then sets off to repeat the routine.

RIDE THE TWO-HEADED BEAST

Played with four children per team. The first two stand, side by side, arms loosely around each others' waists to form the heads and four front legs of the Beast. The third, from behind, bends over and holds on to their arms to form the back and hind legs of the Beast. A fourth rides on the third's back. After one length the four sprint back to the start, switch roles and gallop another length. The relay is completed when each player has been a rider once.

NONSTOP RELAYS

Station the first and last runners of each team at the start-finish line of a 400 m track or other running circuit, and put the other runners at equal distances apart around the loop. Place pylons or other suitable markers at each exchange point. If there are three members per team, there will be two at the start-finish line and the other will be on the opposite side of the field.

Select three to nine runners for each team. The lead runner passes a baton or bean bag to the next runner and stops to wait until it comes around again. Each runner follows the same procedure, and the game can be completed when all runners have returned to their initial positions, or the relay can continue indefinitely.

Having each runner cover more than one lap of accumulated relay 'legs' is desirable for teams of three or four runners who are running longer, slower legs. For example, a well-

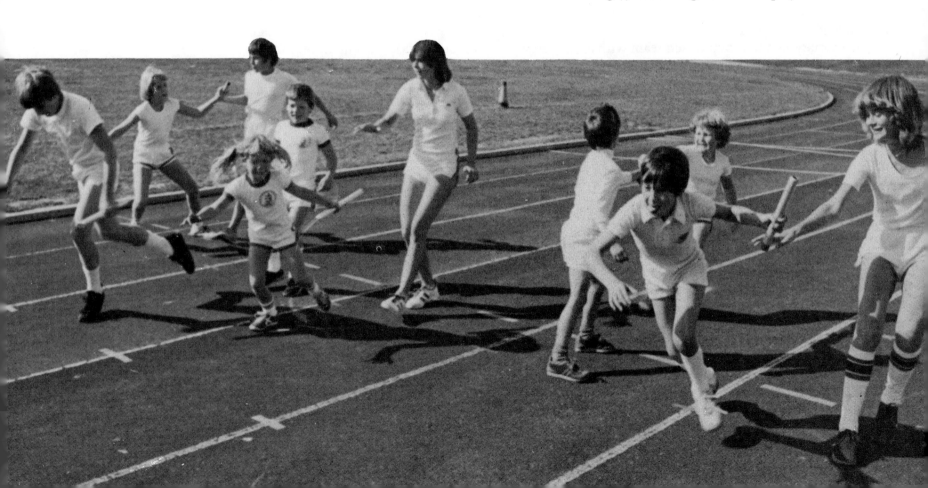

conditioned 13- to 15-year-old on a three-member team on a 400 m track could run 200 m 20 times, equivalent to 10 laps.

One excellent variation of the nonstop relay for older runners is to have each member of a two-member team run one, two, three or four laps each time he or she receives the baton. The rest interval for the waiting runner in this and other well-designed nonstop relays is brief, making for an ideal aerobic workout.

Try this two-member team relay on a 400 m track: when the lead runner has completed 200 m (a half lap), have him or her pass the baton to the partner and then jog slowly across the infield to receive the baton from the incoming partner, who in turn jogs across the field. (See diagram.)

In all nonstop relays, the winner — if it's necessary to declare a winning team — is the first to complete the assignment, or the one covering the greatest distance in a specific time.

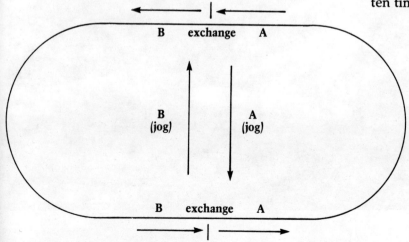

DRAG RELAYS

In this game one partner pretends to be unconscious while the other drags him or her by hands or wrists. After half the distance partners switch roles. Dragging a partner should only be done on a smooth gymnasium floor.

RELAY SCRAMBLE

The first player of a three-member relay team tucks a utility ball or football under his or her arm and runs through a series of obstacles (imaginary tacklers). When the last one is reached, the player turns and throws the ball to the next player, who runs through the obstacles while the first player circles the field to take his or her place behind the last member of the team. The game can be played continuously, each player passing three, five or ten times before the game is halted for a huddle.

RANDOM DISTANCE RELAY

Form teams of three runners and give each team a list of various distances (legs) to be completed as a relay. Team members must run one at a time in a repeating sequence until the entire list of 'legs' has been completed. The list should contain 12, 15, 18 or a greater multiple of 3 legs so that each player runs the same number.

The legs may be run in any order. The best runners will usually do the longest legs. Or, a team may wish to run all the short legs first to build a lead over the other teams and gain a psychological advantage. Of course, the fast starters will have to do the longer legs later in the relay when the other teams will have shorter, faster ones to run.

Teams of older youngsters will want to shuffle their own list, but younger children will probably need the help of an adult to decide in what order they should run the legs. When running on a track outdoors some consideration will have to be given by each team to the problem of where their batons will be exchanged when running a portion of the 400 m.

Here's a sample assignment for teams of older children, say 13 to 15 years, on a 400 m track:

1	leg	of	1600 m
2	legs	of	1200 m each
3	legs	of	800 m each
6	legs	of	400 m each
12	legs	of	200 m each

Here's how a team of runners, A, B, and C, decided to run this Random Distance Relay:

	A:		B:		C:
	A: 200m;		B: 800m;		C: 1600m;
	A: 200m;		B: 400m;		C: 400m;
	A: 200m;		B: 200m;		C: 1200m;
	A: 200m;		B: 400m;		C: 400m;
	A: 200m;		B: 200m;		C: 1200m;
	A: 200m;		B: 400m;		C: 400m;
	A: 200m;		B: 200m;		C: 800m;
	A: 200m;		B: 200m;		C: 800m;
Total	A: 1600m;		B: 2800m;		C: 6800m;

All legs of the relay are completed, but the breakdown shows that the workload was divided by the runners according to ability. A,

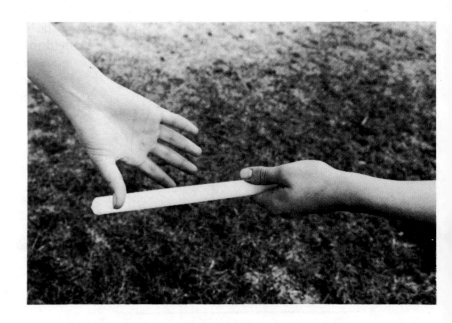

fastest over short distances, ran only 200 m legs totalling 1600 m while C, a distance runner, ran longer legs for a cumulative total of 6800 m. The legs were separated so as to allow a recovery spell between the longest legs.

If Random Distance Relays are run as races, the first team to complete the assignment wins. Idle members of each team will have to use a pencil to check off the legs as they are completed.

Here is a sample assignment for 9- to 12-year-olds on a short indoor lap marked with pylons:

$$6 \times 1\text{-lap circuits}$$
$$5 \times 2\text{-lap circuits}$$
$$4 \times 3\text{-lap circuits}$$
$$3 \times 4\text{-lap circuits}$$
$$2 \times 5\text{-lap circuits}$$
$$1 \times 6\text{-lap circuits}$$

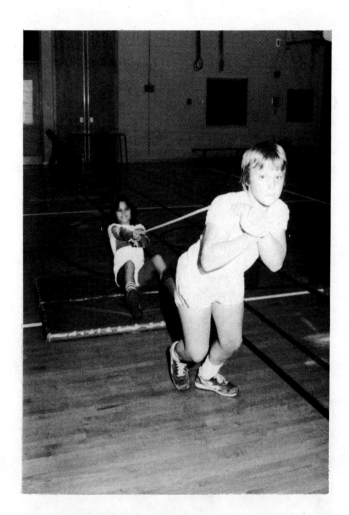

ARMFUL RELAY

For a shuttle relay, have the first of a three-member team pack a hula hoop, medicine ball, Indian club and bean bag one length, deposit the items on the ground and return to the starting line to tag the next member, who then retrieves the goods. Members continue until they have moved the goods back and forth a designated number of times.

As a variation, form piggyback pairs. They can carry more! After one length, switch horse and rider and return with the goods.

TRAILER RELAY

Indoors, one youngster sits on a sack, towel or small blanket and is pulled by a partner with a skipping rope. After one length, they switch roles and return to the starting line.

91

CHAPTER 5
Run for Fun

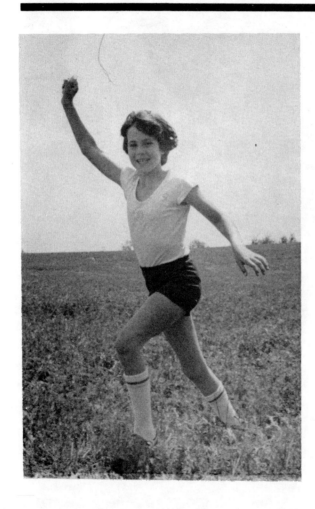

FARTLEK

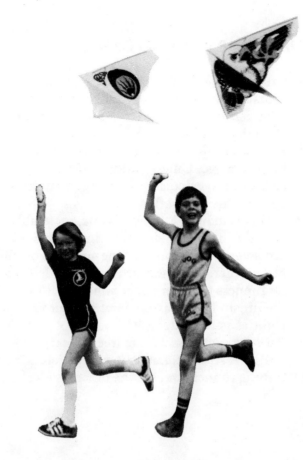

Fartlek, a Swedish word for speed-play, is a natural and creative way to run, particularly appealing to young teenagers. The constant and random change of pace, direction and terrain simulates the running and frolic of frisky animals. Variety banishes boredom, and because the heart rate is raised to near maximum levels and then allowed to recover, Fartlek is an excellent form of exercise.

Advise a well-motivated youngster simply to go for a run and change pace and direction whenever he or she feels like it. The run can last 10 to 40 minutes and cover one to eight kilometres. Small groups can do the same, although freedom is somewhat curbed by having to reach a consensus on changes of pace and direction.

A coach can control the Fartlek workout by running with the youngsters or by confining the group to a small outdoor running area and giving messages by whistle blasts. One short whistle blast could mean 'walk', a long blast 'slow jog', short-long 'rapid pace', and two long 'sprint'. Whistle-Fartlek removes some freedom, but the youngsters remain free to chose where they want to run in the area.

More freedom is permitted in a Fartlek performed by four to eight youngsters, each having a number. Each time the instructor blows the whistle a new leader takes over command of the group and chooses the pace and direction.

Another Fartlek variation is to allow the terrain to dictate the pace. An individual could decide to run up hills rapidly, at a moderate pace on the level, and down hills slowly, or some other combination. In a group, say of four to ten runners, each youngster could take a turn at leading the pace and direction, the lead to change with each change of terrain.

93

HANDICAP RUNNING GAMES

- On a short (40-100 m) indoor or outdoor course, have each participant run one lap for each year of his or her age. Thus, a 13-year-old will run 13 laps, etc.
- Have each run one minute for each year of his or her age. Unless mathematics are employed to calculate and compare runners' speeds, this is a workout only.
- In this Handicap Running Game, preferably for 12- to 15-year-olds, drive the group 5-10 km away from the finish line and drop off the best runner. Then start driving back, letting off runners of lesser talent at points closer to the finish. If your assessment of their various abilities is accurate, it will be a photo finish. For safety, choose a route free of heavy traffic. A straight, flat course in which trailing runners can see the others is ideal.

LOOPS

This running workout is best suited to 13 to 15-year-olds. In a park, large school ground, greenbelt or conservation area, use paths, trees, litter receptacles and other objects as markers outlining two or four circular routes, all starting at the same point. The length of the loops should depend on the age and fitness of the runners. Generally, each circuit should be 250-800 m. Have individuals or groups run each loop in succession, taking a short rest at the starting point after each loop. Depending on the length of the loops, have a runner or group leave the start every three, four or five minutes. (The runner with a slower pace will thus have a shorter rest).

One variation of this excellent aerobic workout is to have pairs working as relay teams. The first runner runs the first loop and tags his or her partner. When the second runner completes the first loop, the rested partner starts the second loop and so on.

Each young athlete should run for a total of 15 to 30 minutes in this workout. That may mean that each runner will run the series of loops more than once.

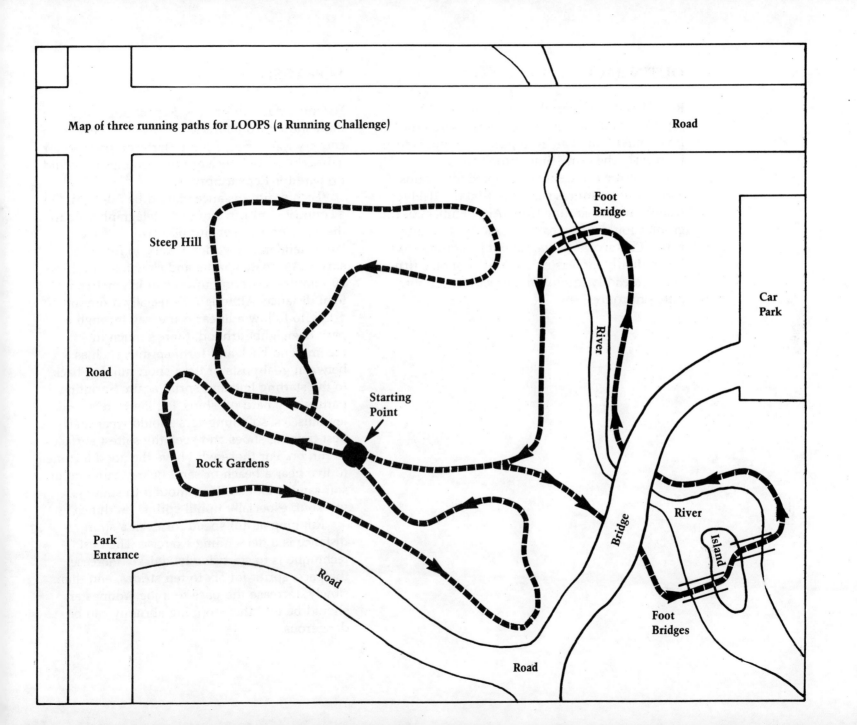

Map of three running paths for LOOPS (a Running Challenge)

Road

Foot
Bridge

Steep Hill

Car
Park

Road

River

Starting
Point

Rock Gardens

Bridge

River

Island

Park
Entrance

Road

Foot
Bridges

Road

OUT'N'BACK

Run for a certain number of minutes, then return to your starting point by the same route. If you have run at an even pace, you will return in exactly the same time it took to run out. This routine can easily be adapted for groups. The trailing runners suddenly find themselves leaders at turn-around time. All members of the group should arrive back at exactly the same time. This workout should not be competitive. By gradually increasing the 'out' distance fitness can be steadily improved. For variety, choose different routes.

REPEAT SPRINTS

For individuals or groups, Repeat Sprints can be done indoors, on a track, on village streets or on country roads. See 'Sprint Starts' on page 83 for a description of how a group of youngsters could prepare for Repeat Sprints.

Each sprint distance should be 50-70 m. On a country road run from one telegraph pole to the next; on a street run past two or three lamp standards. Jog, don't walk, to the next sprint. Alternate sprints and slow jogs for 10 to 20 minutes, covering up to two kilometres in total distance. Although it's usually more interesting to follow a linear route, say through a park or neighbourhood, there's much to recommend back-and-forth sprints, such as between goal posts or up a short hill. Jog back to the starting line and sprint again. Sprinting is particularly hard on shins, leg joints, feet, and leg muscles, so youngsters should wear their best training shoes and seek the softest surfaces to run on. For those who have the good fortune to live near a beach or sand quarry, running in soft sand is an excellent, though frustrating, workout, especially uphill sprints on dunes.

Running at full speed for even a short distance is a demanding exercise. The best technique is to start slowly, quickly increase the pace, sprint for six to ten strides, and then slowly decrease the pace to a jog. Youngsters should be told that stopping abruptly can be dangerous.

Form a chain and invite the lead youngster to run anywhere. Have the chain snake through a series of cones or other obstacles.

In any chain game, if a chain is broken, the players must stop and link up again before proceeding. To discourage breaks, form two or more chains and declare the team that holds together the longest the winner.

Stage a Chain-team Track Meet. Hold events over 100, 400, 800, 1600 metres for teams of 5, 10, 25 and 100 youngsters. Penalties, such as adding three to five seconds to the running time, could be levied against teams in which breaks occur.

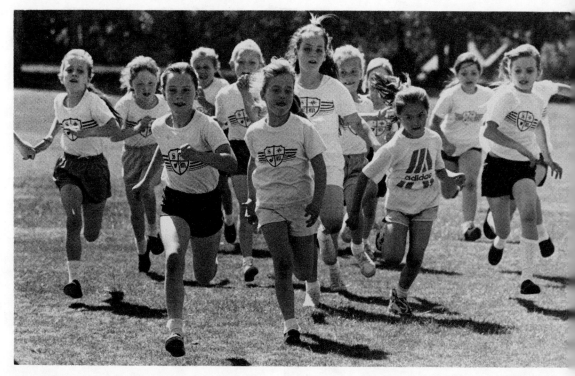

RUNNING CHAINS

Have any number of players join hands or hold a rope to make a chain. Several games and aerobic challenges are now possible.

Form a circle and run in one direction until the instructor blows the whistle, then run the opposite way until the whistle is blown again, and so on.

BEAR RUNS

This running game is suitable for 13 to 15-year-olds, groups of seven to ten youngsters of approximately equal talent. It must be played on open terrain, such as a park, greenbelt or conservation area.

Give one runner a stopwatch and ask him or her to choose a route, straight or otherwise, and run for 45 seconds to three minutes. All others must try to keep up but not get ahead. When the first run is completed, the runners recover by jogging slowly for a time equal to the time they have just spent running. The stopwatch is then given to another runner who chooses another route and sets off, again for 45 seconds to three minutes, while the others follow at pace, if possible.

Eventually, each runner will be leader for one round. This allows each runner to have his input into the workout. Some love hills. Some go crazy on loops, or through rivers. It promotes team unity and spirit and also gives the slower runner some control. Often the runner who is tired and dragging behind suddenly feels good and runs away from the others when he gets the stopwatch in his hand.

UNRAVEL THE CODE

In this entertaining game, the smartest, and not necessarily the strongest or fittest, are often rewarded. The game can be played by individuals or by groups of almost any number. It calls for some advance preparation on the part of the coach.

Each participant is provided with a worksheet similar to the sample shown here. Each of the blanks at the bottom of the sheet represents one letter in a code which will lead to a treasure. The number of each space corresponds to the number of an assignment. When a team completes an assignment it reports the number of the assignment to the group leader, who in return whispers the corresponding letter.

The first team to crack the code, either by completing all the assignments and filling in all the letters, or by figuring it out on the basis of only a few filled-in letters, will find the treasure. No clues are permitted.

The sample sheet outlines a game for two-member teams of 14-year-olds, to be held in a gymnasium marked with large and small circuits. The exercises can be varied to suit the age and ability of the group. In the sample, the code was 'In the bag'.

YOU ARE NOW PARTICIPATING IN
A GAME CALLED "UNRAVEL THE
CODE." READ THESE
INSTRUCTIONS CAREFULLY.

The object of this game is to decipher a code which will lead you to a treasure.

Using this paper and a pencil, work together with your partner, and hide your code from other teams.

At the bottom of this page are 8 blanks. They are to be filled in with letters to form a message, which, when deciphered, will be self-explanatory.

Each time you complete an exercise, you will earn one letter. When you have completed an exercise, report its number to the teacher, who will whisper to you the corresponding code letter. You may do the exercises in any order. In fact, it may be to your advantage *not* to do them in the order shown here.

BEGIN NOW!

1. Each team member must touch all four walls of the gym.

2. Each member must run 10 laps of the large circuit.
3. Do a team total of 30 sit-ups. (e.g., Jean 20, Ranjay 10).
4. Each team member must hop on one foot for one lap of the small circuit.
5. As a *relay*, your team must do two small laps on all fours, stomach-up. This means the second member starts one lap when the first has finished one.
6. Do a team total of 20 push-ups.
7. As a relay, your team must complete 14 large laps, each member running one lap at a time, then exchanging the baton.
8. As a relay and switching places after one lap, your team must do two small laps of wheelbarrow walking.

CODE: __ __ __ __ __ __ __ __
          1 2 3 4 5 6 7 8

LITTLE CIRCLE JOG

Outdoors, designate one station — a dustbin,
piece of clothing, or fixed landmark such as
a tree — for each runner in the group.
The stations should be located in an approximate circle with a 600 m circumference. Have
each runner go to his or her station and then
start the Little Circle Jog. The runner at the first
station jogs to the second station, then both
runners jog to the third. All three continue to
the fourth, the four jog to station five and so on,
until all participants are jogging. The runners
then drop out of the group one by one as they
reach their stations. When the last runner is
back in place, the first begins the Little Circle
Jog again. This is a cooperative running challenge, for the group may not run faster than its
slowest runner. On a 600m circle, six-year-olds
could try one or maybe two circles, while
15-year-olds should be able to jog four to eight
Little Circles.

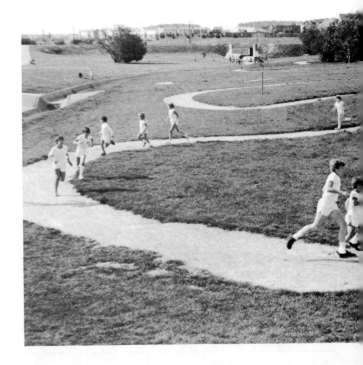

MERRY-GO-ROUND

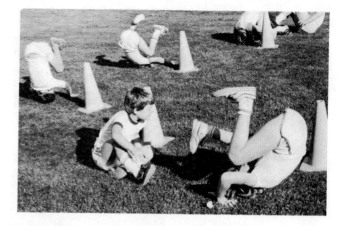

This fun workout is adaptable for groups of any size and is an ideal way to keep a large number of players active and gaining aerobic benefit. It should take place on a 60-80 m track.

The group leader stands in the middle of the circle with a whistle and a watch. Players position themselves around the track. At intervals (timed on the watch), the leader blows the whistle and shouts out a command which tells the player how they must move around the track. Everyone moves in the same direction.

The aerobic value of this activity depends on the choice of exercises, which should be selected so that they suit group requirements and balance strenuous and less strenuous activities.

As an incentive, at the end of a program like the one outlined here, each player can take a turn in the centre with the whistle while the group leader joins the players slogging around the track. Thinking up new movements taxes the imagination almost as much as the exercises tax the muscles.

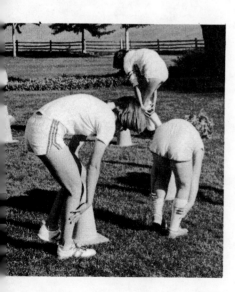

Sample Merry-Go-Round

1. Jog slowly, 1 minute.
2. Walk with high knees, 30 seconds.
3. Walk normally, 30 seconds.
4. Run fast, 15 seconds.
5. Walk slowly, 30 seconds.
6. Repeat exercises 4 and 5, four times each.
7. Walk with hands on knees, right on right, left on left, 30 seconds.
8. Walk with hands holding lower shins, 30 seconds.
9. Jog slowly, 1 minute.
10. Walk backwards, 30 seconds.
11. Walk backwards with long strides, 30 seconds.
12. Run backwards, 30 seconds.
13. Walk backwards, 30 seconds.
14. Run backwards, 30 seconds.
15. Walk forwards normally, 1 minute.
16. Jog slowly, 1 minute.
17. Walk forwards with giant strides, 30 seconds.
18. Touch floor with one hand at each step, 30 seconds.
19. Crab walk, 30 seconds.
20. Repeat exercises 4 and 5, five times each.
21. Walk normally, 1 minute.
22. Jog at moderate pace, 2 minutes.
23. Walk normally, 2 minutes.

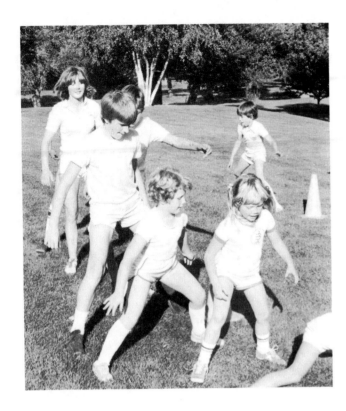

- Hop-Step-Jump. (Both feet, left foot, right foot, both feet, left foot, right foot, &c.)
- Skip to My Loo. (Left foot, left foot, right foot, right foot, left foot, left foot, &c.)
- Hop on right foot, hop on left foot, jump on both feet.
- Piggyback.
- Run with high knees.
- Continuous somersaults (no more than five, to prevent dizziness).
- Roll like a log. (Allow players to roll no more than 5-6 m to prevent dizziness).
- Walk with legs wide apart, bow-legged.
- Walk with right arm and right leg moving in unison in the same direction; the left arm and leg will do the same.
- Walk, clapping hands under lead leg.
- Run, clapping under lead leg.
- Frog hops.
- Walk and move arms various ways — across the body in exaggerated swings; together in large windmilling circles forwards and backwards; reach as high as possible with both hands or alternating arms with each step, make swimming motions (freestyle, breast stroke, butterfly and back stroke); clap hands in front of stomach, behind back and overhead; hold hands of almost straight arms above head moving them from side to side and then forwards and backwards.
- Race walk. (Move as fast as possible, making full use of hips. A simple rule is that one foot must be touching the ground at all times; both can't be off the ground together.)

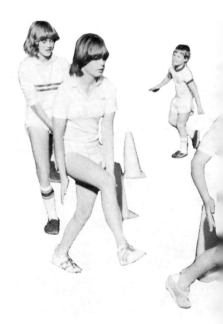

Here are some other mobility modes which can be incorporated into Merry-Go-Rounds. Many can be performed going forwards, backwards and sideways:

- Walk on toes.
- Walk on heels.
- Bear walk. (On all fours, facing down.)
- Walk on outsides of feet.
- Walk on insides of feet.

- Goose step. (Holding straight arms at side of hips, walk with high-kicking straight legs.)
- Walk like a gorilla.
- Walk and then run as if there's a low ceiling. A lower ceiling!
- Crab walk (while raising right leg).
- Bear walk (while raising left leg).
- On all fours, gallop like a horse.
- Do continuous cart wheels.
- Hop on both feet, like repeat standing long jumps.
- Kick right foot high to touch right hand of outstretched arm, repeat with left foot and hand, and so on.

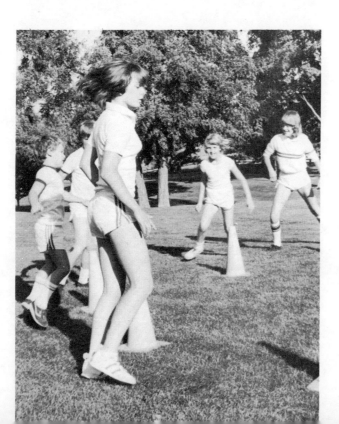

ORIENTEERING

Orienteering was invented in Sweden in 1918. It makes pathfinders out of cross-country runners. It is a sport and recreation that combines running (through familiar or unfamiliar surroundings) and navigating (from a topographical map). It has the same benefits as Fartlek running, and the added advantage — some might say disadvantage — of not knowing exactly how long or how far you will be running. Worrying about whether you are winning, losing, or simply lost, takes the mind off the effort of running.

Orienteering can be a sophisticated sport, but many youngsters, given good coaching, will quickly become adept at reading a map and using a compass.

The standard orienteering course is 3-12 km. Each contestant carries a control card to be punched at the 4 to 15 stations identified by prism-shaped plastic markers along the course.

A simple orienteering contest can be held in school grounds or a local park. The instructor can chalk numbers or symbols on pavements, tree trunks, dustbins, telephone poles, bridges and stones, and make copies of a map or written description giving the location of each station. Contestants run with their maps or description sheets and record the appropriate numbers or symbols as they spot them. The first to return with all the correct symbols marked on the map is the winner.

CHAPTER 6
Aerobic Challenges

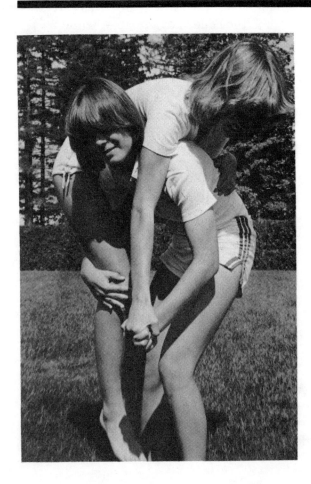

AEROBIC DANCING

Dancing is an excellent way to gain aerobic fitness. Individualistic, creative, uninhibited and sociable, it appeals even to the non-athletic. It is non-competitive, can be done indoors, and needs no expensive equipment.

Volumes have been written on various dance forms, techniques and teaching methods. Among others, disco, modern dance, ballet and square and folk dancing can build aerobic fitness; but the type of dancing and the skill involved are really of secondary importance. The main object is exercise. Dancing to a rapid beat three to five times a week for 15 to 30 minutes at a time could satisfy fitness needs. With rhythmic and vigorous music and positive encouragement from an instructor, even the shyest participants will overcome their inhibitions and dance with abandon.

In recent years, aerobic dancing has been developed to include running, skipping, jumping, hopping, a large number of dance steps, sliding and swinging. Novice dancers are advised to move as they please in time to the music; more accomplished dancers can perform any routine from ballet to modern jazz, from rock to the waltz or polka.

Try starting a co-educational mass aerobic dance programme for your group. Try some disco or even lively country dancing.

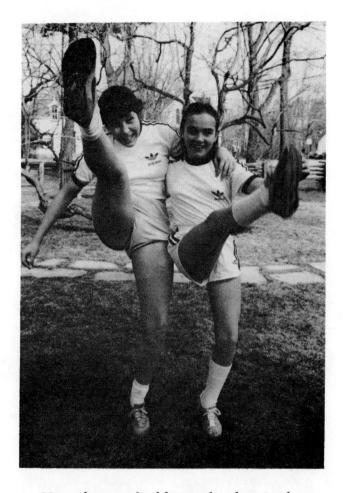

Have the proud athletes who shrug and say that dancing is a feeble form of exercise try some Russian dance steps:

- Cross arms in front of chest, squat, shoot out one foot to the side so leg is straight, and then pull it in as the other foot is thrust out. Repeat until early stages of exhaustion!

105

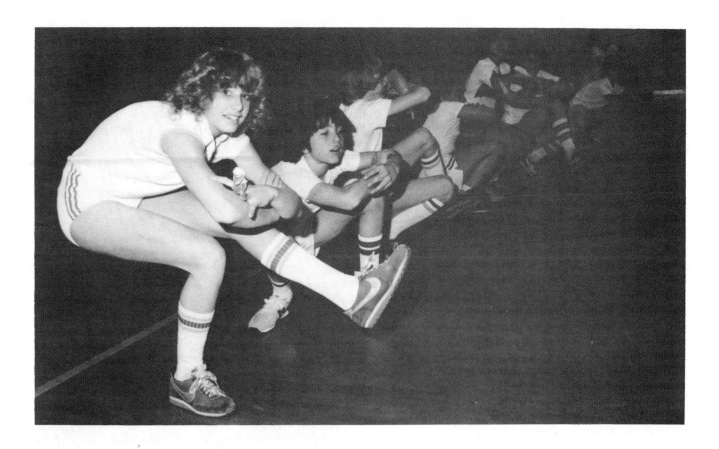

- Try the same step in a partnership. A pair face each other, join hands, squat, and simultaneously extend right then left legs.
- Fold arms in front of chest, finger tips on elbows. From deep squat position, do a sort of leg exchange, first by driving feet forward alternately, and later thrusting feet backwards alternately.
- Stand with feet wide apart, form a 'V' with the arms so that hands are well above head

level, then drop to deep squat on toes with feet close together and arms folded across chest. Return rapidly to the start position and repeat to beat of music.
- In squat position, place right hand on floor at side of right foot, thrust both feet far to the left, and return to the start position. Place left hand outside left foot and do the same move to the right. Repeat.

DUAL TRACK MEET

Stage a 14-event Dual Track Meet outdoors for two (or more!) teams. Each team could have 7, 14, 21, or 28 athletes. Each athlete is to complete in two events. That means that a seven-member team will have one athlete in each event, a 14-member team will have two athletes in each event, and so on.

With mixed teams, say seven girls and seven boys on each, the two sexes could compete together (to save time) but have separate scores. If it is impossible to achieve a 7-boy and 7-girl split, there is no reason why boys and girls should not compete against each other. Strength and skill differences between sexes are almost non-existent in younger children. For older youngsters, teachers may agree to have girls compete against each other in specific events.

Every athlete who finishes an event should earn at least one point. A disqualification or failure to complete an event will result in no points being awarded. Keeping this principle in mind, a variety of scoring tables can be designed. For a Dual Meet in which each team enters two athletes per event, the scoring could be: first, 5 points; second, 3; third, 2; fourth, 1. For a Tri Meet in which each team enters two athletes per event, it could be: first, 10; second, 8; third, 6; fourth, 4; fifth, 2; and sixth, 1.

Below are two categories of events. The first contains short distance and field events, and the second longer running events. Each athlete must compete in one event from each category.

Category One	Category Two
1. 50 m sprint	8. 400 m (1 lap)
2. 100 m	9. 600 m (1-1/2 laps)
3. 200 m	10. 800 m (2 laps)
4. 300 m	11. 1000 m (2-1/2 laps)
5. Long jump	12. 1200 m (3 laps)
6. High jump	13. 1500 m (3-3/4 laps)
7. Shot put	14. 2000 m (5 laps)

Meet Notes:

By refusing to overlap events, this Dual Track Meet with only four or six competitors in each event can be administered by two to four instructors. That is, if the keeping of accurate race times is not a priority!

Follow the order of events listed above. This will allow youngsters who are in two running events time to recover before their second race. To keep the athletes active, warm and interested, sacrifice perfection to efficiency in organizing the meet. Allow only three attempts in the long jump and shot put. Do not let the athletes linger when it is their turn. In the high jump, start the bar at an easy height but raise it by large increments to eliminate the jumpers quickly. In the shot put, 'stake' the first round of throws, and make visual judgements on succeeding rounds.

Inexperienced runners tend to start too fast in distance races. Let them know at the end of

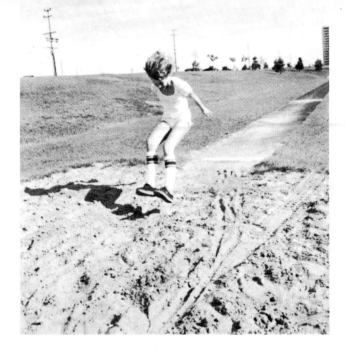

the first half or full lap if they are running a steady pace. If a contestant appears to be straining too hard, pull him or her out of the race. There is no shame in that.

To increase excitement, post the scoring total after each event. Put on an exhibition relay to close the meet. The relay would only be scored to break a tie. Try a continuous sprint relay. Break each team into seven-member relay teams. Place two athletes from each team at the start line and space the remaining five around the track. Mark the exchange points with pylons. Each runner will run 1/6th of a lap and continue to run each time he or she receives the baton. The relay is over when all runners have run six times and returned to their original starting positions.

AEROBATHON

The Aerobathon has a similar format to the pentathlon and decathlon in track and field. Depending on the number of youngsters and leader-helpers, and the available time, select three to ten events for the program. For a full program of ten events, the Aerobathon can be held on successive days.

Odd-numbered events (1,3,5,7 and 9) should be aerobic, with emphasis on running. Even-numbered events, which offer diversion and provide a rest period between the aerobic challenges, should be novelty, strength or flexibility tests. Some sample events are listed below. For other ideas turn to the section on exercises for individuals and choose exercises that are easily measured, such as Squats and Sit-ups.

Considerable planning and organizing may be necessary to avoid long waiting times between events. Have older participants help to officiate.

Score the Aerobathon like a cross country race, giving the best performer in each exercise 1 point; the second, 2; third, 3; and so on. The winner, of course, is the one who accumulates the *lowest* total score. If your group has a wide age variation, the scoring can be handicapped by multiplying each participant's total score by his or her age. For example, a six-year-old with a total of 30 points would achieve a score of 180 (6 times 30). A ten-year-old with the better total of 18 would also score 180 (ten times 18) on the handicapped system. In either system, the contestant with the lowest score is the winner.

Aerobathon events may be chosen from the following suggestions, but many other events, with the exception of hurdles, pole vault, discus and javelin, can also be used. The exceptions either require too much skill or present a hazard, particularly to younger participants.

The distances here are merely recommendations. Lengthen or shorten them according to the fitness level of the group.

Sprint

Have only two or three youngsters run in any one heat so that accurate split times can be made. Award places by times; don't have heats and finals.

6-10 years	50 m
11-15	100 m

Middle Distance

6-7 years	200 m
8-9	250 m
10-11	300 m
12-13	400 m
14-15	600 m

Long Distance

6-7 years	400 m
8-9	600 m
10-11	800 m
12-13	1200 m
14-15	1500 m

Sprint Backwards

6-10 years	20 m
11-15	50 m

One Foot Hop

Hop on right foot one half the distance recommended below, then hop the second half on the left foot.

6-10 years	30 m
11-15	50 m

Timed Short Slalom Run

See description on page 39.

Obstacle Course

See description on page 56.

Incline Run

If possible, incorporate stair or hill running into the Aerobathon.

Strength events

See Fitness Test on page 123 for description of how to measure Push-ups and Sit-ups.

Shot Put

Outdoors, use the smallest available shot put for all ages. Indoors, use a medicine ball or the smallest indoor shot put. Indoors, have all competitors try to hit a bare wall from a short distance. Each round, have participants throw from a point farther from the wall, and eliminate those who are unable to hit it. This avoids the time-consuming chore of measuring throws.

Chin-ups

Not appropriate for very young players.

High Reach
Tape a measuring-tape to a wall. Have the contestant stand flat-footed next to the wall and reach as high up the tape as possible. Then have him or her jump as high as possible, touching their finger tips to the tape. Each competitor's score is the difference, in centimetres, between standing and jumping reach.

Long Jump
Do regular running long jumps outdoors if a pit is available. If not, or indoors, do a standing long jump. Give each participant two attempts, and record the best effort.

High Jump
Give competitors only two chances to make a height. To speed up the competition, don't allow "psyching-up" time between jumps, and raise the bar several centimetres after each round.

See overleaf for photocopiable Sample Score Sheet

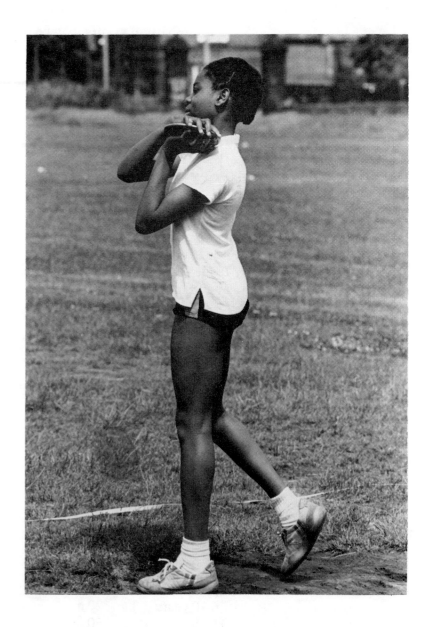

AEROBATHON
[Sample Score Sheet]

Competitor's Name	1 res	1 pl	2 res	2 pl	3 res	3 pl	4 res	4 pl	5 res	5 pl	6 res	6 pl	7 res	7 pl	8 res	8 pl	9 res	9 pl	10 res	10 pl	Total	Age	Handicap Total	Place

Events (result = res) (place = pl)

Permission is granted to photostat this for school use

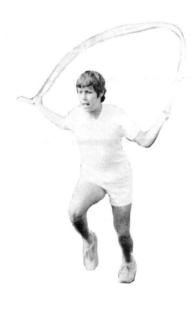

AEROBIC CIRCUITS

Circuit training is a favorite of track coaches because it's so adaptable to specific aerobic, strength and skill goals. The activities can be designed for various age levels.

Make several stations around the gymnasium or playing field, each having a printed description of the exercise to be performed there, and any necessary equipment. Avoid having more than three players at a station at any one time during the activity: no one should have to wait in line for equipment.

Not all exercises need to be done at the station itself. For instance, Station Six may have an instruction to run four laps of the gymnasium. Don't prescribe exercises, such as forwards and backwards running on the same track, that could lead participants to interfere with each other.

Explain how to perform each exercise before circuits are started. Put one to three players at each station and instruct them to move in the same direction to their next stations.

Circuits can be competitive. For example, the winner could be the player who is first to complete one circuit, or the player with the highest number of exercises completed in four, six or eight minutes. But the competitive element may contribute to having the exercises too hastily or improperly performed. Players should be praised more for skill and thoroughness than for speed.

The number and combination of routines are limited only by imagination. Some suggested Circuit ideas follow:

Big Circuits (11 to 15 years)

Station No.	Exercise	Repetitions
1.	Half-squats	15
2.	Skipping	100 turns of the rope
3.	Push-ups	10
4.	Knee slaps	50
5.	Rest 1 minute	
6.	Down and Out	5
7.	Leg Exchanges	20
8.	Chin-ups	20
9.	Step-ups	20
10.	Sit-ups	10

Little Circuits (6 to 10 years)

In gymnasium, mark an outer and inner lap, 5 m square.

Station No.	Exercise	Repetitions
1.	Jog	4 big laps
2.	Crab walk	1 little lap
3.	Arm Circles	10 one way; 10 the other way
4.	Run	2 big laps
5.	Twister (standing)	10
6.	Walk holding backs of thighs	1 little lap
7.	Run backwards	1 big lap
8.	Hop on right foot	1 little lap
9.	Hop on left foot	1 little lap
10.	Mule kicks	20

Partner Circuits (11 to 15 years)

In a gymnasium, mark outer and inner laps. The figure in the repetitions column gives the number of repetitions for each partner. The same partner should start each new exercise. For relays, partners take turns in succession. By eliminating the carrying exercises, Partner Circuits can be adapted for younger players.

Station No.	Exercise	Repetitions
1.	Jog relay	3 times 3 big laps
2.	Piggyback	1 big lap
3.	Wheelbarrow	1 little lap
4.	Sit-ups (partner holds ankles)	20
5.	Up the Creek	40
6.	Piggyback Heel Raises	10
7.	Leapfrog	1 little lap (total)
8.	Ski-sit	1 little lap
9.	Piggyback Squats (quarter knee-bend)	10
10.	Running relay	4 times 2 big laps

Circuit Training

The following comprehensive circuit programme is for a 15-year-old aiming to build overall fitness. To gain full benefit, the youngster who doesn't participate in other activities should do this workout three or four times a week. For those wishing to improve their fitness for sports, once or twice a week will be sufficient.

Start at Level One and perform the exercises in the order shown. That is one circuit. For the first week or two, do the Level One circuit only once in each workout. After that, take a five-minute rest after the first circuit and do it a second time. Set a time goal; when two circuits can be achieved comfortably in less than target time, move to Level Two and do two circuits per workout until sufficient progress is made to graduate to Level Three. For variety, change the order of the exercises.

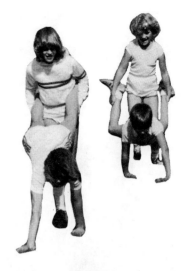

Exercises	Level One	Level Two	Level Three
(Warm-up)			
Lean a Little (4 positions)	20 sec. each pos.	20 sec. each pos.	20 sec. each pos.
Heel Raises (both feet)	20	20	20
Jog (Slowly)	4 min.	4 min.	4 min.
Swivel Hips	5	5	5
Bent-Knee Sit-ups	3 × 12	3 × 16	3 × 20
(Circuit)			
Push-ups	3 × 5	3 × 7	3 × 10
Chin-ups (on bar)	3 × 3	3 × 4	3 × 5
Skipping	100 rope turns	150 rope turns	rope turns
Half Squats	20	30	40
Run on Spot (high knee)	1 min.	1 min. 30 secs.	2 min.
Step-ups (40 cm)	25	30	35
Book Jumps (30 cm)	8	10	12
Leg Exchanges	20	30	40
Down and Out	5	8	12

CYCLING

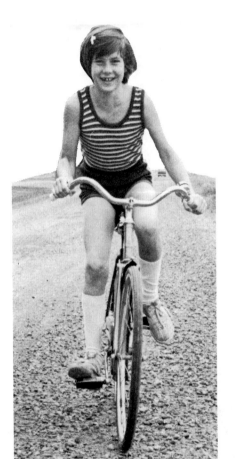

Whilst accepting that it is not always easy to organise, cycling can be a rewarding outdoor and adventurous activity.

Cycling is a complex sport, best suited to older teenagers and adults, but younger children love to ride. Take advantage of their enthusiasm to teach them good safety habits, riding technique and proper bicycle maintenance and repair.

Cycling can be aerobic exercise, but the cyclist has to work hard to gain as much benefit as a runner. On a flat smooth surface, the cyclist has only to overcome friction and wind resistance to maintain a good speed. Uphill cycling is much more difficult and quickly raises the heart rate. For this reason, repeat hill climbing is an excellent cycling workout.

Before taking part in cycling activities, carefully instruct youngsters on where, when and how to ride to avoid hazards lurking on the roads.

Make certain each bicycle is in good working order and seats are placed at a comfortable height. Most seats are too low to allow an effective extension of legs. Give youngsters a short lesson on how to pedal correctly. "Ankling" means the heel is slightly below the level of the pedal when it is at the 12 and 6 o' clock positions. When travelling in groups, cyclists should go in single file along the side of the road with the traffic flow and remain a safe distance apart. They should carry water bottles on warm days and a small amount of money in their pockets for emergencies, such as an urgent need for food or to make a phone call home.

Always keep both hands on the handle bars.

Have your group plan its own tour, encourage them to choose the least busy roads. The distance of the trip should depend on the age of the youngsters and the time available. Some ambitious 15-year-olds will cycle up to 80 km on a morning's outing, although that distance is not recommended for younger children or those with only a moderate interest in fitness. Select an unusual route with things to see and do (a picnic, a visit to a farm, or other rural location, or to a park to hold an Aerobic Games Track Meet). That will help take the riders' minds off their cycling effort. Have parents assist, either by trailing in cars or riding along.

One sport that has gained popularity among some fitness extremists is uphill cycle races. On some steep hills, the real test is not how fast you can cycle, but whether you can actually make it to the top without having to get off and walk.

AQUAEROBICS

Most watersports, from breaststroke lengths to water polo, improve overall strength and aerobic fitness. Clocking up freestyle lengths of the swimming pool is an excellent training workout, but unless you're very dedicated to the sport, it can be a little dull. These Aquaerobics will provide variety.

WATER VOLLEYBALL

Water Volleyball should be played in a pool of uniform depth. Water should be at about waist level, so players can easily stand on the bottom. The top of the net should be 1 m above the surface of the water. All the rules of regular volleyball apply. The resistance of the water increases the aerobic fitness.

WET PURSUIT

In a four-sided pool, one swimmer is stationed at the centre of each side. At the signal, each swims in the same direction, chasing the one ahead. Each swimmer must touch the centre point of each side before continuing. When one swimmer overtakes another, the tagged swimmer drops out of the game. Continue the game for two minutes or until only one swimmer is left, whichever occurs first.

WATER RELAYS

In the simplest form of water relay, team members swim in sequence. No swimmer may enter the water until the previous swimmer has touched the end of the pool: false starts will incur time penalties. All swimmers may use the same stroke, or different strokes may be used in successive legs.

Many of the suggestions in the section Races and Relays can be adapted for swimmers. Retriever Relays are well suited for swimming pools. Team members swim the length of the pool, climb out, retrieve or deposit some object (sticks, floats, balls and tyres are all appropriate) at the far end, re-enter the pool and swim back to the start line. Following swimmers repeat the routine, until the specified goal has been accomplished.

WATER SCRAMBLE

Suitable for large groups, this game requires a number of floats — equal to the number of players. Write a number on each float, and throw the floats into the pool so that they are fairly evenly distributed. Each player is then assigned a number and must try to find the float whose number matches his own. As players pick up floats bearing the wrong numbers, they are permitted to throw these into another area of the pool, the object being not only to find your own number but to prevent other people from finding theirs.

TIME TRIALS

Holding time trials in running, swimming, cycling, cross country work and other endurance sports is an excellent way to motivate youngsters in the off season. Because young athletes can wait for ideal weather conditions, and the competition is against the clock, not against other people, time trials are a true measure of how well they are prograssing at their chosen endurance sport.

Time trials are not only part of an interval training programme. A swimmer, cyclist or track athlete on long distance training may use a time trial to check short distance speed. Or a trial may be held for healthy youngsters who have been improving their fitness through a variety of sports disciplines. A swimmer may run a mile, and a runner cycle 20 km in a time trial.

Because time trials are stressful, participants must be free of medical problems, have a proper warm-up, and be supervised and advised to stop if they suddenly feel ill.

The following time trial description is for young track athletes, but some principles can be applied to other sports. (Different from most other time trials, cyclists must ride several metres apart during a time trial to avoid drafting, the advantage of having wind resistance reduced by the presence of the rider in the front.)

Time trials to measure the aerobic capacity of young runners should be at least 600 m. (Time trials over shorter distances are a greater measure of sprinting ability and anaerobic capacity.) A moderately fit but untrained and unskilled 14- or 15-year-old might try a time trial distance of 1200-3000 m. Distances in excess of these may cause undue fatigue, blisters and discouragement.

Time trials should be held on 400 m tracks because they are flat, free of obstacles and standard. (A youngster could thus run a trial on a track while on holiday in another area or indeed country.) An athlete will often gain a false impression, either of dramatic personal improvement or of a discouraging loss of endurance, after taking part in a time trial held off-track, where the distance is estimated or measured by a car trip meter.

Set target times for each lap, and advise the youngsters to run an even pace. The tendency will be for them to start too fast, not fully appreciating the distance to be run. Best performance times are achieved by even pace. If a youngster starts much too fast or slow, postpone the time trial, preferably to another day, and try again.

116

INTERVAL RUNNING

Most competitive track runners and even cross country runners believe that interval training is one of the quickest methods of obtaining top aerobic fitness. Some precocious 13 to 15-year-olds may benefit from non-rigid interval training, but it's not recommended for younger children. What is described here is for youngsters who have more than a casual interest in sport and fitness. Principles of interval running can easily be applied with success to swimming, cycling and cross-country work.

Interval (running) training can be done almost anywhere, but a 400 m track with its exact measurements and level surface is ideal. Interval training can be boring, so the instructor should plan some off-track workouts. Youngsters should taste the joy of running wild through the woods or clambering up a hillside.

Young people can gear their interval programme to the sports in which they wish to participate. Those in sports such as football which require short bursts of speed should run shorter distances, and middle-distance runners, longer distances. Volumes could be filled with varieties of interval programs. Interval training has four basic components: 1. The distance to be run; 2. The number of times the distance should be run; 3. Pace; 4. Rest or recovery.

1. Distance to be Run.

Greatest gains in aerobic fitness are made by running one and a half to three minutes at a pace that will raise the heart rate to 75 to 85 per cent of its predicted maximum, usually 150 to 170 beats a minute.

A 13- to 15-year-old should be able to run 350 m or more in one and a half minutes and 700 m, more or less, in three minutes. Therefore, most of the distances run in the interval program should be 300-800 m. Some longer and shorter interval runs will also be useful.

2. Number of Times to Run the Distance

A rule of thumb for determining the total distance to be run in a workout is to multiply the 'goal' distance by two or three. So, if the goal is to run 1600 m in six minutes, the workout distances should be 3-4 km, not including the distance jogged in warm-ups, cool-downs and during recovery periods between interval runs. For such a goal, the interval workout could consist of 8 to 10 times 400 m or 5 to 7 times 600 m. Interesting interval programs combine various distances and paces. Many of the workouts outlined below start with longer distances and step down to shorter distances. This allows the body time to adjust to the pace.

3. Pace

Training pace should be approximately the same as that required to complete the goal successfully. For training distances in excess of one quarter of the goal distance, the pace should be slightly slower than goal pace. For training distances that are shorter, the pace should be slightly faster than that needed to achieve the goal. (For example, a youngster training for 1 600 m in six minutes should run 400 m in one and a half minutes. Pace for shorter distances will be faster, and vice versa.)

Here's a sample chart of paces for a youngster seeking to run 1 600 metres in 6 minutes:

Distance	Time
100 m	16 seconds
200 m	38 seconds
300 m	62 seconds
400 m KEY PACE	**90 seconds**
500 m	1 minute 58 seconds
600 m	2 minutes 25 seconds
800 m	3 minutes 20 seconds
1000 m	4 minutes 15 seconds
1200 m	5 minutes 15 seconds

If a youngster can't run at goal-pace for one quarter of the goal distance, then the goal is too ambitious and should be reduced. On the other hand, if the youngster finds the pace too slow, an early date should be set for a time trial.

4. Recovery

There are four ways to measure the rest period between runs:

- Jog or walk a part or the whole distance that has just been run. A youngster running 400 m might jog slowly for 400 m or walk 200 m before starting the next 400 m run.
- Time the rest period, say, equal to the time it takes to run the training distance. A one-and-a-half-minute 400 m run would be followed by one and a half minutes of rest.
- If training with others, the rest period could be the time it takes a partner to run a training distance. This workout is similar to a continuous or non-stop relay.
- Monitor the pulse. When the runner's pulse drops below a certain level, say 100 to 120 beats per minute, then he or she is ready to start running the next distance. Taking the recovery pulse is more difficult but it's the best way to determine the optimum rest period. It usually takes longer to recover as the workout progresses. Monitoring the pulse permits longer rest and doesn't force a youngster to run tired. It may require several workouts to learn how to read the pulse quickly and decide what rate indicates that recovery has been achieved.

Sample Programme

The following is a sample programme for a youngster who is not a competitive track athlete but wishes to improve his or her athletic ability, aerobic capacity, and health. It's based on a goal of running 1600 m in six minutes, a rather ambitious objective for an average 13 to 15-year-old. Each workout begins with a warm-up. These should include ankle rotations, heel raises, a light 800 m jog, hamstring stretches, and abdominal and upper body exercises. See the section on individual exercises for other warm-up ideas. After following this programme for three weeks, have the young runner stay away from the track for one or two weeks before returning to another three-week interval programme.

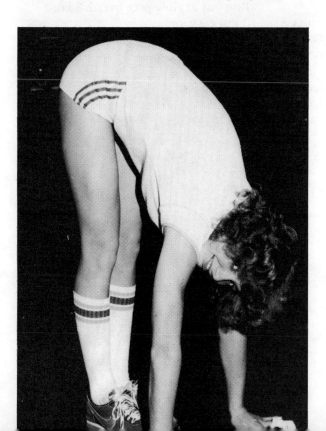

First Week

Monday (Off track)	Jog 3-4 km, constantly changing pace, over grassy surface.
Tuesday (On track)	Six laps of gradually increasing pace. The first 400 m should be about 2 minutes and 20 seconds and the last 400 m in about 1 minute and 45 seconds. Four times 400 m in 90 seconds each, followed by a suitable rest period. Run-out, a slow jog of 2 to 3 laps.
Wednesday (Off track)	Jog 3-4 km on soft surface Six times 30 m sprint up a short hill Run-out
Thursday (On track)	Two times 400 m in 90 seconds each 200 m in 38 seconds 600 m in 2 minutes and 25 seconds 200 m 600 m 200 m Two times 400 m in 90 seconds each
Friday (Off track)	1600 m slow jog or complete rest
Saturday (On track)	Time Trial. (Ask the runner to run at a 90-second 400 m pace. If after the first two laps the runner is too slow, he or she has misjudged the pace or is not ready for the six-minute 1600 m. Abandon the trial and try again in three to five weeks.)
Sunday (Off track)	Run at easy pace for 5-8 km

Second Week

Monday (Off track)	Run 5 km on a hilly course
Tuesday (On track)	3 laps (1200 m) in 5 minutes and 15 seconds
	2-1/2 laps (1000 m) in 4 minutes and 15 seconds
	2 laps (800 m) in 3 minutes and 20 seconds
	Four times 200 m in 38 seconds each
	Run-out
Wednesday (Off track)	5 km jog
	Four times 100 m sprints on grass
	Run-out
Thursday (On track)	2-1/2 laps in 4 minutes and 15 seconds
	2 laps in 3 minutes and 20 seconds
	600 m in 2 minutes and 25 seconds
	400 m in 90 seconds
	Six times 200 m in 38 seconds each
	Run-out
Friday (Off track)	1600 m slow jog or complete rest
Saturday (Off track)	Eight to twelve times run up slope of 140-200 m
	Run-out
Sunday (Off track)	Run at easy pace for 6-10 km

	Two times 400 m in 90 seconds each
	Four times 80 m sprints
	Run-out
Wednesday (Off track)	Jog 3-6 km constantly changing pace
Thursday (On track)	600 m at gradually increasing pace
	Two times 400 m at gradually increasing pace
	300 m in 62 seconds, (100 m interval jog)
	200 m in 38 seconds, (100 m interval jog)
	100 m in 16 seconds (3 to 5 minute rest)
	Repeat the 300-200-100 sequence
	Run-out at slow pace over 2-3 km
Friday (Off track)	3 km easy jog
Saturday (Off track)	5 km easy jog
Sunday (Off track)	6-10 km jog

Third Week

Monday (Off track)	5 km of repeat sprints and jogs
	Walk for 3 to 5 minutes after each kilometre
Tuesday (On track)	Two times 1000 m in 4 minutes and 15 seconds each
	Two times 800 m in 3 minutes and 20 seconds each

PULSE PACING

Teach youngsters to find their pulse by placing three fingers of one hand on the thumbside of the wrist of the other hand. Another pulse can be found on either side of the Adam's apple under the back of the jaw bone. Take this pulse on only one side of the neck. Do not press hard, or the blood flow to the head may be slowed.

Because pulse rates are closely related to oxygen consumption, they are a fairly good measure of fitness. Given a certain workload, such as jogging or running upstairs, the lower the heart rate, the better the fitness. However, like most instant indicators of fitness, do not accept pulse rates as an absolute. Great individual differences have been recorded without any obvious explanation.

Note: the following routine is for 14- and 15-year-olds. The pulse rate figures given here are meaningless for younger children.

Maximum rates in young children are high, and both the resting and maximum rates tend to get slower as children grow older. A standard 'training' aerobic pulse rate for 14- to 15-year-olds is 140 to 150 beats per minute. Instruct your group to jog on a flat surface for two minutes and then have them stop, find their pulse, and count it for only six seconds, and multiply by ten to get their jogging pulse. It is important to get the pulse reading immediately,

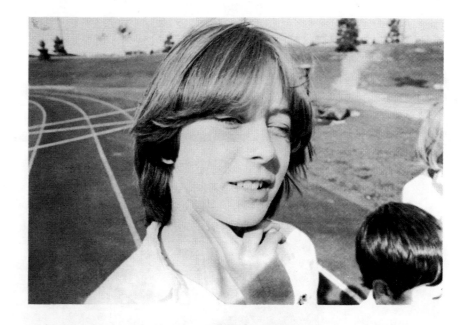

or it will slow down. If runners have rates above 150, ask them to slow down on the next two-minute jog; for those with rates lower than 140, urge them to speed up for the next two minutes. Runners should run evenly until they establish a 'training pace' in which their hearts are beating 140 to 150 times per minute.

Explain that for training purposes, it is more important to have a good training pulse rate than running a fast pace. Some will have to run fast to raise their heart rates, while others will achieve a rapid pulse while jogging.

This Pulse Pacing programme can also be done while swimming, stair stepping and cycling.

CHAPTER 7

How Fit Are You?

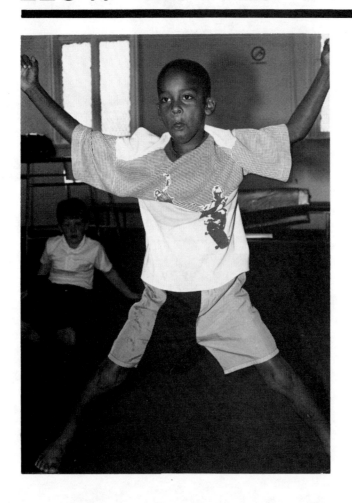

Fitness Test

This simple test offers an unrefined indication of a youngster's abdominal and upper body strength, aerobic capacity, and flexibility. Use the chart on page 126 to record scores, and compare the scores achieved by members of your group with each other and with the averages provided on the chart. These were gained by testing 200 children in a typical school.

Demonstrate each exercise before starting the test.

Speed Sit-ups

Lie back, knees bent and together, and interlace fingers behind head. A partner or adult tester straddles the lower legs, pressing feet to the floor and holding the back of the calves, just under the knees. Keeping hands behind the head throughout test, the participant must sit up, touch elbows to knees, and return to touch shoulders to the floor. Each time elbows touch knees the partner counts one repetition. For youngsters who can't do one Sit-up, allow no compromise on technique. It's simply an indication that the child's abdominal strength is inadequate. This test should last for 30 seconds.

Push-ups

Participants under ten should do Push-ups from the knees, all others should do ordinary Push-ups. Whether from the knees or by the regular method, participants should hold their bodies straight and rigid, touching the floor with their entire bodies and then rising to a straight arm position with each repetition. This test should last for 20 seconds.

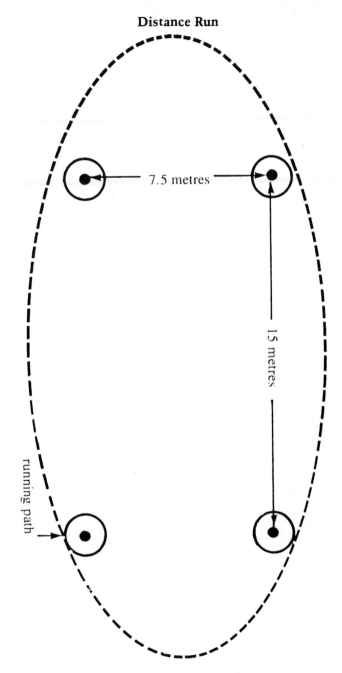

Distance Run

7.5 metres

15 metres

running path

Distance Run

The measure of the standard lap, for which norms are given below, is 45 m, but participants will run 10-15 m further, since their route around the markers is oval. There is thus no point in comparing their times with those achieved over equal distances on regular 400 m tracks. Have participants run one lap for each year of their age, six-year-olds running six laps and so on. Although this test can be performed outdoors, an indoor environment has been used here because it's more universally available. The circuit should be marked off with four pylons in the shape of a rectangle, the long sides 15 m and the short 7.5m.

Seated Straight-Leg Reach

Have participants sit straight-legged on the floor and press bare feet against the vertical side of a low box or stack of books supported by a wall. Each child will reach slowly forward, beyond the toes, if possible. A ruler fixed to the top of the box or books can be used to measure the 'plus' (beyond toes) or 'minus' (short of toes) distance of the reach. The ruler should be touched with the fingers of both hands at the same time.

FITNESS TEST

	Age	15	14	13	12	11	10	9	8	7	6
Sit-ups (30 sec.)	boys	27	27	26	25	24	22	20	18	14	9
(Repetitions)	girls	23	23	23	26	23	20	19	18	12	7
Push-ups (20 sec.)	b.	18	18	17	17	16	16	16	16	15	8
(Repetitions)	g.	9	10	11	16	16	16	15	15	15	10
45 m. run (x age)	b.	3:10	3:02	2:52	2:42	2:34	2:16	2:02	1:49	1:40	1:34
(Minutes:seconds)	g.	3:42	3:30	3:22	2:52	2:48	2:35	2:18	2:04	1:47	1:38
toe touch (+ or −)	b.	+2	+1	+1	−0	−0	−0	+1	+1	+1	+2
(Centimetres)	g.	+8	+5	+5	+3	+3	+5	+5	+5	+8	+8

NATIONAL CURRICULUM KEY STAGE GRID

Exercise	Page No.	Key Stage 1	2	3	4
Double LegThrusts	11		*	*	
Down and Out	11	*	*	*	*
Knee Tuck Jumps	11		*	*	
Ground Loops	12		*	*	*
Compass Circles	12		*	*	*
Hoop-de-Hoop	12	*	*		
Leg Exchanges	13		*	*	
Mule Kick	13		*	*	
Squats	13		*	*	*
One Legged Squat	14		*	*	*
Stationary Starts	14			*	*
Step Ups	14	*	*	*	*
Poses	16	*	*		
Straddle Hops	16	*	*		
Lunge	16	*	*		
Twister	16		*	*	*
Frog Hops	17	*	*	*	
Push-Ups	17			*	*
Sit-Ups	18		*	*	*
Roll Up and Tuck	18			*	*
Two-Point Crouch	18		*	*	
Wall Walk	19	*	*		
All Over Stretch	19			*	*
Imitations	20	*	*		
Floor Hip Stretch	20		*	*	
Lean a Little	20	*	*	*	
Goin' Nowhere	20		*	*	
Hurdle Stretch	20		*	*	*
High Hurdle Stretch	21		*	*	
Stretch and Slouch	21	*	*	*	*
Swivel Hips	21	*	*	*	*
Don't Kick Me	22			*	*
Lots of Squats	22		*	*	
Partner Ski-Sits	22		*	*	*
Back-Up-Me	23		*	*	
Partner Pull-Ups	23		*	*	
Up the Creek with a Partner	23		*	*	*
Partner Chin-Ups	24		*	*	
Piggyback Exercises	25			*	*
Capture the Flag	27		*	*	
Bulldogs	28	*	*		
Some Bulldog Variations	29		*		
Scramble	29	*	*		
Flamingoes	30		*	*	
Hangar Flying	31		*	*	
Loony Ball	32	*	*		
Scurry	32	*			
Keepers Weepers	33		*	*	*
Musical Hoops	34	*	*		
Retriever Trials	34	*	*		
Run the Gauntlet	35	*	*	*	*
Victory Ball	36		*	*	
Team Frisbee	37	*	*		
Hula Hoops	39	*	*	*	
Short Slalom Run	39	*	*		
Aerobic Chance	40		*	*	
Poison Pull	41		*	*	
Net the Fish	41	*	*		
Heavy Catch	41		*	*	
Gruesome Twosomes	42		*	*	
Lions and Tigers	44	*	*		
Bull-Rings	44		*	*	*
Elimination Hop	46		*	*	
Lift and Laugh	46		*	*	
Four Walls	47		*	*	
Mat Clash	47		*	*	
Surprise	48	*	*	*	*
Piggyback Games	49			*	*
Basketball for Children	52		*	*	*
Basketbrawl	52			*	*
Aerobic Hopscotch	53		*	*	
Hockey for Children	55			*	*
Frisbee Tennis	55		*	*	*
Leapfrog	56		*	*	
Obstacle Course	56			*	*
Forward Passes	58			*	*
Buck Passing	58			*	
Horsemen of the Apocalypse	59			*	
Soft Lacrosse	59			*	*
Touch Rugger	60		*	*	
Singles Volleyball	60		*	*	*
Tug of War	61		*	*	
Three Men in a Tug	61		*	*	

NATIONAL CURRICULUM KEY STAGE GRID

Exercise	Page No.	1	2	3	4
Team Tug of War	62	*	*	*	
Individual Tug of War	62		*	*	*
Skipping	64	*	*	*	
Ropey Routines	67			*	*
Soccer	68		*	*	*
Mini Soccer	69		*	*	*
One-Pass Soccer	69		*	*	
Hand Soccer	70		*	*	
Crab Soccer	70		*	*	
Ball Tag	71	*	*		
Hang Tag	72		*	*	
Line Tag	72	*	*		
Aerobic Immunity Tag	72		*	*	
Polo Tag	72		*	*	
Snow tag	72	*	*	*	
Team Tag	73		*	*	
Water Tag	73	*	*	*	*
Optional Tag	73		*	*	
Bean Bag Tag	75		*	*	
Double Agent Tag	75		*	*	
Always It Tag	75		*	*	
Chain-Gang Tag	75		*	*	
Five Points Down Tag	75		*	*	
Companion Tag	76	*	*		
Cuddle Tag	76	*	*		
Bee Sting Tag	76	*	*		
Three's A Crowd Tag	76		*	*	
Tandem-Tag	76	*	*	*	
Reversed Partner Tag	76		*	*	
Shadow Tag	76	*	*		
Posse Tag	77	*	*		
Frozen Tag	77		*	*	
Imitation Tag	77	*	*		
Flamingo Tag	77	*	*		
Sprint	79	*	*	*	*
Bear Walk	79	*	*		
Crab Walk	79	*	*		
Both Arms, One Leg	80			*	*
Bunny Hop	80	*	*		
Crooked Walking	80	*	*		
Gawky Run	80	*	*	*	
Hop-Along	80		*	*	

Exercise	Page No.	1	2	3	4
Seal Slide	80	*	*		
Worm	80	*	*		
Elephant Walk	80		*		
Sticky Foot	81		*	*	
Rigid Legs	81	*	*		
Partner Hops	81		*	*	*
Bums Rush	82	*	*	*	
Backwards Hop	82	*	*		
Broken Foot	82	*	*		
Heavy, Man, Real Heavy	82	*	*	*	*
Devil Take the Hindmost	83	*	*	*	
Sprint Starts	83	*	*	*	*
Sideways Skip	84	*	*		
Dribbling	84		*	*	
Basketball Shooting Race	84			*	*
Relays	85	*	*	*	*
Stick-with-It Relay	86	*	*		
Holding Hands	86		*	*	
Under-Over Relay	86		*	*	
A Relay Potpourri	86		*	*	
Three-Legged Games	86	*	*	*	
Construction Relay	87	*			
Add and Subtraction Relay	87		*	*	
Stick Hop Relay	87		*	*	
Ride the Two-Headed Beast	87			*	
Non-Stop Relays	88	*	*	*	*
Drag Relays	89		*	*	
Relay Scramble	89		*	*	
Random Distance Relay	90		*	*	
Armful Relay	91		*	*	
Trailer Relay	91		*	*	
Fartlek	93		*	*	*
Handicap Running Games	94			*	*
Loops	94				*
Out 'n' Back	96			*	*
Repeat Sprints	96			*	*
Running Chains	97	*	*	*	*
Bear Runs	98				*
Unravel the Code	98				*
Little Circle Jog	100	*	*	*	*
Merry-Go-Round	101		*	*	*
Orienteering	103				*

NATIONAL CURRICULUM KEY STAGE GRID

Exercise	Page No.	Key Stage 1	2	3	4
Aerobic Dancing	105			*	*
Dual Track Meet	107		*	*	*
Aerobathon	108	*	*	*	*
Aerobic Circuits	112	*	*	*	*
Cycling	114		*	*	*
Aquarobics	115		*	*	*
Water Volleyball	115			*	*
Wet Puruit	115			*	*
Water Relays	115	*	*	*	
Water Scramble	115	*	*	*	
Time Trials	116				*
Interval Running	117			*	
Sample Programme	119				*
Pulse Racing	121			*	*
Fitness Tests	123		*	*	*

Foulsham Educational also publish the standard work

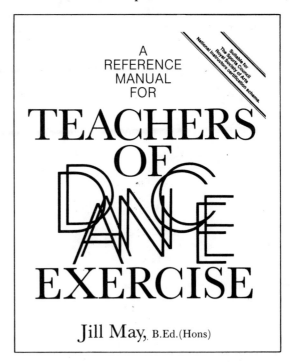

A REFERENCE MANUAL FOR

TEACHERS OF DANCE EXERCISE

Jill May, B.Ed.(Hons)

Suitable for
The Sports Council
The Royal Society of Arts
National Instructors certification scheme

Recommended by The Sports Council, The Royal Society of Arts, and for use with the National Instructor's Certification schemes.

The National Curriculum syllabus for Key Stage 4 requires a knowledge of basic exercise principles F.I.T.T., and the practical application of those skills in an exercise programme. The components of Cardio-Vascular Fitness, Muscular Strength and Endurance and Flexibility are an essential part of this exercise programme.

All of these key components are to be found in this manual, with practical advice on composing your own personal programme for health-related fitness.

ISBN: 0-572-01472-4